Stretching for Health

Stretching for Health

Your Handbook for
Ultimate Wellness, Longevity,
and Productivity

JERRY WEINERT and JILL BIELAWSKI

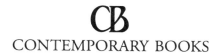

CONTEMPORARY BOOKS

Library of Congress Cataloging-in-Publication Data

Jerry Weinert.
     Stretching for health : your handbook for ultimate wellness, longevity, and
productivity / Jerry Weinert and Jill Bielawski.
         p. cm.
     Includes index.
     ISBN 0-8092-2436-4
     1. Stretching exercises—Handbooks, manuals, etc. I. Jill Bielawski. II. Title.
  RA781.63 . B53 2000
  613.7—dc21   00-22657
                                                             CIP

Cover design by Jennifer Locke
Cover photograph copyright © David S. Robbins/Stone
Interior design and illustrations by Precision Graphics Services, Inc.

Published by Contemporary Books
A division of NTC/Contemporary Publishing Group, Inc.
4255 West Touhy Avenue, Lincolnwood (Chicago), Illinois 60712-1975 U.S.A.
Copyright © 2000 by Jerry Weinert and Jill Bielawski
Printed in the United States of America
International Standard Book Number: 0-8092-2436-4

00 01 02 03 04 05 VL 19 18 17 16 15 14 13 12 11 10 9 8 7 6 5 4 3 2 1

To those who have read, used, been inspired by, and given great feedback about our earlier publication, Head to Toe: A Manual of Wellness and Flexibility,

and to

Valeria W. Bielawski, Jenn Brooks, Annie Campbell, Mark Cochran, Bella Eibensteiner, Betsy Lancefield, Karen Lunda, Aaron Mattes, Joey Tanner, and Stephanie Weinert.

Special thanks for support, patience, feedback, and encouragement to Chris Gans.

Contents

Foreword

Quality of life is determined by its activity.
—Socrates

Optimum health and well-being are attained and maintained through a balanced program of nutrition, exercise, and rest. Often the body becomes imbalanced, resulting in sickness or injury. Muscle weakness and inflexibility are present in a high percentage of the adult population.

Stretching is intended to be a simple, painless method of preparation for movement. Many techniques tend to aggravate the tissues and result in immediate pain or later soreness. There is a unanimous agreement that flexibility is specific; that is, the degree of range of motion is specific for each joint. For example, a flexible shoulder does not ensure a flexible ankle, and range of motion in one hip may not be highly related to range of motion in the other hip.

In therapy, stretching is an important modality for regaining flexibility. Flexibility coupled with strength helps develop body fitness, posture, and symmetry, and it assists in alleviating pain and increases relaxation.

The potential benefits of flexibility are virtually unlimited. Circulation is improved, oxygen is delivered faster and more efficiently, the lymphatic system is aided to work with greater effectiveness, nutrition is delivered to tissue, and cells are no longer ischemic.

Active-isolated stretching is about incorporating specific, gentle, relaxing movements to invigorate the circulatory, respiratory, and neuromuscular systems to help release stress. It is a technique that respects how the body physiology works. "No pain, no gain" is a dangerous philosophy and should not be part of tissue enhancement.

Well-chosen stretching exercises can help the individual regain lost range of motion. Consistent flexibility training will help maintain tissue health and help prevent or alleviate pain or injury. Along with the aging process, there is frequently loss of flexibility, strength, and stamina. A well-constructed stretching program can help to restore those qualities.

In his book *Guide to Turning Back the Clock,* Robert Arnot, M.D., explains that active-isolated stretching is the first technique he found that improved his flexibility without the pain and frustration produced by many other techniques.

The book you are about to read is a guide to enhance the health of young or old, healthy or deconditioned, including those who are weak, injured, postoperative, or suffering from neurological deficits.

—AARON L. MATTES

Aaron L. Mattes received his Bachelor of Science from Wisconsin State University–Superior in 1970, majoring in physical education. Mattes received his Master of Science from the University of Illinois at Urbana-Champaign, in 1972, with special emphasis in kinesiology and exercise therapy. His experience encompasses more than 125,000 hours in instruction, rehabilitation, athletic training, adapted physical education, sports medicine, and preventive programs. He is a registered kinesiotherapist, a licensed massage therapist, and a certified rehabilitation administrator.

Preface

Challenges make you discover things about yourself that you never really knew. They're what make the instrument stretch—what make you go beyond the norm.

—Cicely Tyson

Have you ever thought about "cleaning up your act" through better wellness and exercise choices, but when you checked it out found the material written about this field overwhelming? Do you have a condition that limits your activities or creates considerable discomfort? Does your work or recreation require repetitive motion? Are you uncomfortable and therefore less productive in your daily routines than you would like to be? If you answered yes to any of these questions, then this book was written for you—in clear terms and a conversational style.

We started out to write a client or patient education brochure about stretching, but we soon saw this project needed a broader scope. A scan of available information revealed that most books on this subject were geared toward the therapist or athlete, were too technical, or were limited in scope. Few publications combine wellness and self-help principles with a flexibility-based fitness program.

Both authors of this book are massage therapists with a background in complementary medicine, education, rehabilitation, and fitness. We wanted to answer the questions our clients asked us most frequently, because your questions about how, why, and what to stretch take a significant amount of therapy time. So does addressing health and wellness behaviors and identifying cause-and-effect patterns that contribute to painful conditions.

We hope this book will reinforce the teaching and recommendations of your therapy or health assessment session.

The first five chapters offer a concise overview of general health and wellness concerns. They describe how your activities can create ill health or persistent pain. We provide you with suggestions about how to begin adopting a healthier lifestyle. And we give special consideration to the reality of our modern culture and busy lifestyles. We include descriptions of the most common conditions that create discomfort and immobility, along with self-help measures that can help you gain control over your daily activities.

Chapter 6 is the central focus of the book. It features a detailed and easy-to-understand approach to the active-isolated method of stretching. Jerry Weinert was introduced to active-isolated stretching by Aaron Mattes in Nashville, Tennessee. Jill Bielawski received her introduction from Aaron in Miami, Florida. We both have found, more than any other method, the active-isolated approach to be effective at safely increasing our own full-body flexibility, and we've used these techniques successfully with our clients. Besides describing a full-body flexibility routine that takes approximately forty minutes, we have created "seven-minute stretch breaks" for different regions of the body. This is one more acknowledgment of the reality of the busy lives we lead.

At the end of Chapter 6 we've included a section that covers the questions our clients ask us most frequently. Following that chapter is a glossary that defines technical terms.

In addition to being a self-health guide and patient/client education tool, we believe this book is a valuable resource for the physician, physical therapist, and massage therapist. But, primarily, it's an important starting point for those willing to select a path toward improved health and wellness.

The secret of getting ahead is getting started.
—Sally Berger

Introduction

If life means movement and death means nonmovement, then . . . more movement means more life and less movement means less life. . . . A diminished capacity for movement is equivalent to diminished life.

—Thomas Hanna

Flexibility is the key to health and wellness both literally and symbolically. As you embark upon a path of comfortable stretching and flexibility practice, your body becomes better toned, better balanced, and moves more easily. A flexible body makes for a flexible mind. Regular practice of flexibility exercises helps you tune into the breath and the overall status of the body. It can be meditative and may help you to be focused. As your awareness of yourself as a physical being increases by understanding the various options for fluid movement, so will you enhance your mental awareness by understanding the numerous options and choices available to you for problem solving or life management. A higher level of wellness also results from a less rigid and more flexible lifestyle. Improved flexibility allows us to listen to our bodies and to hear what they may be saying, rather than forcing some unreasonable activity or agenda on them. The same principle works for our emotional, mental, and spiritual selves. If we are flexible enough to listen to what others are saying and what inner needs we may have, rather than remaining on automatic pilot, we will develop better emotional, mental, and spiritual balance, less stress, and a greater level of health and wellness.

The attainment of physical and mental flexibility is a gradual process that requires daily practice. True change in a posture or an attitude does not happen overnight. It has taken many years for each one of us to develop our various functional and dysfunctional habits. Thus, it may take months or even years to assimilate new, healthier, and better balanced physical posture and mental attitudes. As your body shifts toward improved awareness, new insights will continue to creep into your conscious mind that will help bring balance to your whole physical, mental, emotional, and spiritual being.

Typically, we come into this world as open, willing, able, and ready creatures. Most of us are born relatively unscathed, with unlimited potential for growth. As we progress through the infancy and toddler stages, we begin to develop our cognitive beliefs of how the world is for us—secure or insecure, fun or frightening. Our opinions are often formed during this time based upon our experience with our parents or caregivers. Their parenting skills, contentment with life, and general level of happiness, for the most part, determine whether our early childhood experience is positive or negative, expansive or contracted. Mental flexibility, or lack thereof, gets a start in early life. Similarly, our physical agility seems to be at its peak during the preschool years. Once we begin sitting at a school desk five hours daily, our bodies' flexibility starts a decline. Various childhood traumas (falls, abuse, emotional insults) further impact our ability to be expansive and flexible. Since we are creatures drawn to comfort, our boundaries continue to contract with each trauma. Movement becomes more limited with each trauma in order to avoid pain or further injury. To expand beyond the limits set by our physical comfort or early established belief system requires an actively conscious process of our whole being. Thus, an effort to become more flexible requires rebuilding neglected physical functions, reframing mental and emotional beliefs, and reconnecting to others who are sharing this amazing human experience.

Chapter 1

Wellness

Flexibility . . . more than physical fitness, it's a state of being!

A wise man should consider that health is the greatest of human blessings.

—Hippocrates

Simply defined, wellness is quality of life. It includes dimensions of physical, social, emotional, intellectual, spiritual, and even occupational well-being. Wellness is a way of living more fully; enjoying physical health, energy, and vitality; and finding a sense of meaning in work, family, and community. It is a behavioral style that allows you to feel good more often—without harm to yourself or others. Adopting this behavioral style may reduce your risk of premature death and/or disability. While modern Western medicine has accomplished incredible surgical and pharmacological feats in treating various traumas, illnesses, and diseases, it has all but forgotten centuries old natural and behavioral methods to treat and prevent infirmity. During the past fifty years, medical education has essentially ignored the prevention of disease. It views health as the absence of disease. We view health as striving toward high-level wellness. To quote W. H. Auden, "Health is a state about which medicine has nothing to say."

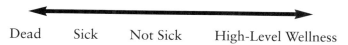

Dead   Sick   Not Sick   High-Level Wellness

A person's health may fall anywhere along a continuum. Most of us go through life being not sick. This is a far cry from high-level wellness. With high-level wellness, there is more congruity between our physical activities, personal relationships, nutrition, occupations, spiritual beliefs, and mental and emotional outlooks. With more balance and satisfaction in these areas, the body moves away from the "not sick" part of the continuum. When the body is a more fully aligned organism, immunity to disease is enhanced, and there is more resilience in dealing with the various daily stressors.

If your behavior moves toward the high-level wellness end of the continuum (regular exercise, no tobacco use, eight hours of nightly sleep, a balanced diet, good stress management practices, satisfying relationships, defensive driving, a gratifying job), then it seems to take quite a large "assault" to move back toward the sick end of the continuum. If you are living on the high-level wellness end and catch a flu bug, you are more likely to be sick only a day or two instead of the week or two manifested by "everyone else."

While it is not always possible to find the "perfect job" or the "perfect relationship," you can take steps to gain control over your life. The key is to learn how to direct your own behavior patterns to minimize those that create pain in your life and maximize those that create pleasure, enjoyment, productivity, cooperation, and collaboration. This might mean making choices to begin an exercise program, learn healthier cooking routines, or enter into counseling to improve relationships. It could mean eliminating habits that are unhealthy (smoking, lack of sleep, too much caffeine or sugar) and honestly examining parts of your life that may cause stress.

This book will address some basic factors you can implement to move closer to a wellness-oriented lifestyle. The next section offers ideas on lifestyle changes. Remember, changes can be difficult and come slowly. As trite as it may sound, some changes are better than none. So identify a couple of activities you've been putting off and pursue them. Gradually add other activities over the next weeks or months. Old patterns have a strong hold at times, so a slip back to the old ways is not reason to forget the whole thing. Any "failure" is a learning situation, and with each situation you learn how to do it better. Be understanding and forgiving of yourself and reintroduce the more desirable healthy behaviors. A wellness-oriented lifestyle is a wonderful gift to yourself. The rewards of increased vitality and self-satisfaction are close at hand. Enjoy the journey!

> *Human beings, by changing the inner attitudes of their minds, can change the outer aspects of their lives.*
> —William James

Lifestyle Change Strategies

Turning over a "new leaf" and making the choice to change a lifelong pattern may seem a bit overwhelming. It may be so overwhelming for many that they decide to forget it for fear of failure or not knowing where to begin. As we suggest throughout the book, begin with small changes and, as these become part of your life, add new ones.

It is important to identify the behavior you want to change and have a good reason for wanting to change it. Does the behavior cause you pain? Does it interfere with your sleep? Does it make you feel stressed? Does it affect your relationships with your family or friends?

Once the behavior is identified and the reason for wanting to change is clear, then set a long-term goal as to how you would like to see your life look with this behavior changed. Now plan the first step, one of many short-term goals. It may take many steps to accomplish the long-term goal, and it may take many months. Remember, it took you years to get to where you are now. Changes do not happen overnight. If you find that you have failed to meet one of your many short-term goals on the way to the larger goal, this can also be a success. Think about it. Most successes don't "just happen." They often occur because you've learned from a previous failure and decided to change. Failure can be a success because it is a lesson that provides more insight to the process. Often major changes in lifestyle happen in a "two steps forward, one step back" pattern. As long as there's forward momentum, congratulations are in order!

It is also important to identify potential barriers to your goal and how you will deal with each. We chose, consciously or unconsciously, a particular behavior, habit, or pattern because it brought some sort of satisfaction. So, in the process of lifestyle change, resistance will arise. The body and psyche have grown accustomed to the behavior. How will you manage this resistance without throwing away your good intentions?

Social support is another necessary factor to facilitate lifestyle change. Enlist the moral support and assistance of a family member or friend. How can they help you achieve your goal? Discuss your progress regularly to keep your goal in your active consciousness and as a means to receive objective feedback on your progress. Rewards are good motivators! Behavior modification programs for children, which reward good behavior, are known to be effective for reinforcing desirable behavior. Variations of these programs work very well with adults too. In this case, you are the one in control. You identify the desired behavior and the time frame for its accomplishment, and you also get to set the reward. Try assigning point values to meeting minor goals. After you accumulate so many points, reward yourself. This is a good opportunity to set a reward system that encourages a healthy lifestyle. With this in mind, a banana split would not be an appropriate reward. As a reward, consider receiving a massage, going to a concert, or taking a minivacation.

Reevaluate your short-term and long-term goals after three weeks, six weeks, three months, and six months. Write these dates on your calendar. If you find your initial goal was unrealistic, modify it so that you feel good about your work toward this goal. Change requires a conscious and active commitment. Enroll yourself in a plan designed by you in order to benefit you. Remember, you have everything to gain.

> *There are two ways of meeting difficulties. You alter the difficulties or you alter yourself to meet them.*
>
> —Phyllis Bottome

Good Sleep

Sleep is a necessary component for the body to thrive and function on the wellness end of the continuum. Without adequate rest, it's difficult for the body to replenish important hormones and energy reserves.

The nervous system has a remarkable tolerance for short-term sleep loss. With temporary sleep loss, there is minimal effect on performance. Most individuals can maintain usual performance with 60 to 70 percent of normal sleep. While performance may not be compromised with temporary sleep loss, there still are consequences. Moderate sleep loss creates irritability and fatigue.

Long-term sleep loss falls into the category of insomnia. There are three classifications of insomnia:

1. Sleep-onset insomnia—difficulty falling asleep, defined by an average of thirty minutes per night to fall asleep.
2. Sleep-maintenance insomnia—difficulty staying asleep; that is, waking up in the middle of the night and staying awake longer than thirty minutes. Early-morning awakening with inability to fall back asleep is another type.
3. Poor quality of sleep—a decrease in normal sleep for more than a few days can impair performance and cause mood disturbances.

Factors that cause insomnia include the following:

- stress
- caffeine, alcohol, or drug consumption (alcohol may facilitate ease of falling asleep, but the quality of sleep is impaired, and there is difficulty staying asleep)
- inadequate exercise
- depression
- unrealistic sleep expectations
- inappropriate scheduling of sleep
- trying too hard to sleep

Stages of Sleep

During normal, restful sleep, you progress through five stages of sleep in a ninety-minute period.

> Stage 1 is the lightest stage, marking the transition from wakefulness to sleep. If awakened in stage 1, you would probably say you weren't sleeping. Apparently this is the stage that artist Salvador Dali is reported to have never progressed from. It's said that he would rest every few hours holding a pen in his hand. As soon as the pen fell to the floor, he had gotten all the sleep he needed and was up again for a few hours. You be the judge if you think this might have created a "mood disturbance."
>
> Stage 2 is the first "true" stage of sleep, marked by light sleep from which you can easily be awakened.
>
> Stages 3 and 4 are known as delta sleep, the deepest stages of sleep. It is difficult to be awakened from delta sleep.
>
> Stage 5 is REM (rapid eye movement) sleep or dream sleep. Virtually all dreaming occurs during REM sleep. REM is a lighter stage of sleep.

During the first part of the night, delta cycles are longer and REM cycles are short. As the night progresses, delta sleep decreases and REM sleep increases. More repair and restore hormones are released with subsequent REM cycles. Also, dreaming becomes more active the more REM cycles you complete. Thus, you are doing your body a favor by getting at least four REM cycles (four ninety-minute cycles = six hours). While a ninety-minute cycle to move through all the stages of sleep is not exact for everyone, you may find that awakening after a complete cycle will produce a more satisfied feeling of rest. In other words, try planning your sleep so that you awaken after four to six REM cycles (six, seven and a half, or nine hours). If you awaken feeling very groggy, you may have been in the middle of delta sleep.

Tips for Good Sleep

Towson University researcher Karla Kubitz states: "When the body temperature begins to cool down, which occurs late in the evening, it may be a signal that it's time for us to feel sleepy. . . . Exercise may help people sleep by warming up our bodies, which then cool down as a result." A similar effect is related to a hot bath. The bath raises the body's temperature, bringing relaxation to the muscles, and the subsequent cooling may trigger sleep.

Many of us believe that certain foods, and when we eat them, affect how well we sleep. While this belief may aid our sleep patterns, there is little research on the subject. Several studies indicate that there is no food or time of eating, in relation to sleep, that improves one's sleep.

Here are some tried and true tips for solid sleep:

- Get regular exercise, earlier in the day.
- Avoid caffeine (which is found in, in addition to coffee and tea, soda, coffee yogurts and ice cream, and some pain relievers).
- Avoid alcohol close to bedtime.
- Take a hot bath near bedtime.
- Go to bed and awaken at the same time every day.
- Use the bed mainly for sleeping. Read or watch television in a chair.

Good restful sleep allows us to have a more balanced perspective on the events of our lives. It can make us more productive, happy, and pleasant in our relations with others. Sleep not only helps our mood and psychological outlook, it is important on a cellular and physical level, giving our tissues a chance to restore and function optimally.

Relationship of Oxygen to Wellness

Oxygen is married to wellness, and they are inseparable partners. It is only at death that they part. Certain environmental conditions and personal behaviors create conflict between the two, which can result in pain, discomfort, illness, and loss of function. Does this mean you have to manage yet another high maintenance relationship? Not quite. But it is necessary to nurture this relationship if your goal is movement toward high-level wellness.

The essential principle supporting the recommendations in this book is to increase nutrient availability to the tissues, that is, to create an environment within your body that allows more oxygen to bathe the organs and muscles. The more oxygen available, the more vital and healthy we become.

Why do you have muscle pain? There are a number of possible reasons, but the underlying problem is ischemia (lack of oxygen). Most people have heard of cardiac ischemia, commonly known as angina, which usually results in chest pain. This is due to narrow coronary arteries, which carry oxygen-rich blood to the heart muscle. Because they are narrow (from cholesterol buildup, for example), they can't deliver as much oxygen, and this creates pain. This is true for any muscle in the body. If the blood flow is restricted from a tight muscle or spasm (like a kink in a garden hose), less oxygen will be available. With less blood flow and less oxygen getting to the muscle, there's also a buildup of metabolic waste products that can't get out of the muscle. These waste products contain acids that create even more irritation in the tissues. Massage, stretching, reducing stress, and aerobic exercise all help muscles to relax, thus allowing more oxygen into the tissues and flushing waste products out of the tissues.

We have little control over the air we breathe. Thus, in a rural wooded area without industrial smokestacks, the air is cleaner and richer in oxygen. Conversely, in heavily populated and industrialized cities, the air is polluted with a cocktail of chemicals that leave less room for oxygen. Ever wonder why the country folk live longer? Breathing polluted air also creates more free radicals in the body. Free radicals are a byproduct of oxidation and speed the aging/deterioration process. Since we have little control over the air we breathe, it makes sense to try to do something to give your body a better chance to utilize oxygen. You can control this by reducing environmental stressors, such as secondhand smoke, allergens, noise, and other noxious stimuli.

The first and foremost activity you can control is to stop smoking if you smoke and to stop being around smoke, even secondhand tobacco smoke or campfire smoke, for example. Where there's smoke, there's carbon monoxide, an invisible, odorless gas that can be deadly. Carbon monoxide displaces oxygen. That is, if carbon monoxide is around, the body will pick it up and leave oxygen behind.

So, the picture is forming. You're tense and have an old injury that is guarded with tight muscles. You don't have time to exercise and are too busy to have much relaxation time. You happen to be a smoker and wonder why you're irritable and in a lot of pain. Take a look. You're not giving your body a chance to let in much oxygen. But there are some choices that can change this scenario.

Aerobic activity is one of the best methods to increase the oxygen distribution throughout your body. This doesn't need to be done in a sweaty health club with loud music and people wearing skin-tight matching outfits. The way the body uses oxygen as its energy source is through rhythmic and continuous movement, which includes activities like walking, cycling, and swimming. We will develop this idea more thoroughly in our chapter on fitness.

Numerous massage techniques are designed to loosen tight, constricted muscles, relieve spasms, and alleviate tension. Tightness and tension limit the amount of oxygen available to your muscles. The less oxygen, the more pain you experience. Massage is also an excellent means to help rid the muscles of metabolic waste and infuse oxygen-rich blood back into those tissues, thus reducing pain.

Stress creates tension. Muscles become tighter and organs malfunction. Hundreds of books have been written on how to manage stress. A few of the simple suggestions in this book are a good place to begin. A regular flexibility program is a great way to ease stress. Stretching not only lengthens and loosens muscles, it can be a form of meditation and centering. The simple act of doing something that may move you to a higher level of wellness is a good stress-management tool.

These are some of the ways to keep the love light burning between oxygen and wellness. And, as supple, movable muscles are an important part of this couple feeling forever young, their relationship will be even further nurtured with an eating plan full of great wholesome food.

Chapter 2

Nutritional Considerations

The soul needs to be fattened .... Good food for the soul includes especially anything that promotes intimacy: a hike in nature, a late night conversation with a friend, a family dinner, a job that satisfies deeply, a visit to a cemetery. Beauty, solitude, and deep pleasure also keep the soul well fed.

—Thomas Moore

Food is the fun part (who doesn't like to eat?), and perhaps the most challenging. Most eating patterns become set by the time we are old enough to be living away from our childhood home. Any shift away from our customary foods can be a threat to our sense of security, comfort, and cultural belonging. Food is ritual. Food is reward. Food is relief from depression. Food is celebration. Food is memory. Food is nutrition. Food is sharing. Overall, food is associated with all parts of our physical, mental, emotional, and spiritual well-being. How to choose healthier foods and maintain the integrity of your association with food's pleasures is the challenge. Flexibility around exploring new tastes, textures, and traditions is the fun part.

Eating healthily does not mean feeling deprived. Healthful and delicious foods are abundant. A change of pattern requires you to reframe what, why, and how you deal with food and to be conscious and creative about healthy choices.

What Is Nutrition?

Nutrition is the relationship of foods to the health of the body. Proper nutrition means that all the essential nutrients, carbohydrates, fats, proteins, vitamins, minerals, and water are supplied and utilized in adequate balance to maintain optimal health. Changing these nutrients into smaller, simpler substances for ready use within the body is the process of digestion.

The main activity of digestion is to break down

- carbohydrates into simple sugars (glucose),
- proteins into amino acids,
- and fats into fatty acids and glycerol.

People today probably have more information about what is "good" for them than ever before. Yet, we are growing fatter and less fit. Obesity is a significant contributing factor to numerous health problems, including diabetes, back and other musculoskeletal pain, and various digestive disturbances. (According to the Metropolitan Life standardized tables, obesity is defined as being above ideal body weight by 20 percent or more.) High-fat foods, low fiber intake, and lack of fresh fruits and vegetables all contribute to various cancers. Heart disease, the leading killer in the United States, is very highly correlated to imbalanced or improper nutrition.

Good nutrition is essential for normal organ development and functioning; for normal reproduction, growth, and maintenance; for optimum activity level and working efficiency; for bolstering the immune system to resist infection and disease; and for the ability to repair bodily damage or injury. No single substance will maintain vibrant health. While some nutrients are known to be more important in certain bodily functions, they are interdependent and synergistic with all other nutrients in order to maintain homeostasis or balance.

Components of Food

Carbohydrates, fats, and proteins are the primary sources of energy to the body because they supply the fuel necessary for body heat and work. Their fuel potential is expressed in calories, a term that signifies the amount of chemical energy that may be released as heat when food is metabolized. (A calorie is a unit of heat. It takes 1,000 calories to raise a kilogram—one quart—of water one degree Celsius.) Therefore, foods that are high in energy value are high in calories and vice versa. Fats yield approximately 9 calories per gram, or 225 calories per ounce, and carbohydrates and proteins yield approximately 4 calories per gram, or 115 calories per ounce. Fats are the slowest burning fuel. They are the coal. Proteins burn almost twice as quickly as fats. They are the hardwood. Carbohydrates burn quickly. They are the softwood and kindling. Other important components of food include minerals, vitamins, and water.

Carbohydrates

Carbohydrates are the chief source of energy for all body functions and muscular exertion and are necessary to assist in the digestion and assimilation of foods. They provide us with immediately available calories for energy and also help regulate protein and fat metabolism.

Carbohydrates are broadly classified as simple and complex. Simple carbohydrates are sugars such as those in honey and fruits. Sucrose, or table sugar, is a double sugar, but it is not nearly as complex as a starch. Complex carbohydrates are made up of chains of sugars. Complex carbohydrates include the starches found in potatoes, whole grains, pasta, and bread.

Unrefined, natural carbohydrates (veggies, fruits, whole grains, and potatoes) burn like softwoods in the fireplace. In addition to being rich sources of vitamins and minerals, these foods provide a steady burning fire that will last many hours.

Refined carbohydrates (table sugar, sucrose) are like kindling in the fireplace, providing a burst of flame that is soon gone. They are immediately absorbed into the bloodstream. This creates the short-lived "rush" you experience after eating a chocolate bar or drinking a soda pop. As quick as they give the rush, they also provide a comparable letdown.

Ingestion of refined carbohydrates can lead to many disorders. High intake results in overstimulation of the pancreas that can wear out this important gland, creating diabetes. Overindulgence can also lead to hypoglycemia, a condition in which the body is no longer able to metabolize sugar properly. A diet high in refined carbohydrates contributes to a feeling of fatigue and clouded thinking. It will also lack essential vitamins, minerals, and fiber. Cravings for sweets are best satisfied with fresh fruit.

Fats

Fats, or lipids, are the most concentrated source of energy in the diet. In the fireplace analogy, fats burn like coal, the hardest and slowest burning fuel. They contain twice as much energy per gram as the other fuels—proteins and carbohydrates. In addition to providing energy, fats act as carriers for the fat-soluble vitamins, A, D, E, and K. By aiding in absorption of vitamin D, fats help make calcium available to body tissues. Fats prolong the process of digestion by slowing down the stomach's secretions of hydrochloric acid. Thus, fats create a longer lasting sense of fullness after a meal. Fat deposits cushion, protect, and hold vital organs in place. Fat also is the body's insulation against environmental temperature changes.

The substances that give fats their different flavors, textures, and melting points are known as the fatty acids. There are two types of fatty acids, saturated and unsaturated. Saturated fatty acids are those that are usually hard at room temperature and, except for coconut oil, come primarily from animal sources. Unsaturated fatty acids, including monounsaturates and polyunsaturates, are usually liquid at room temperature and are derived from vegetable, nut, or seed sources, such as corn, safflowers, sunflowers, and olives.

Monounsaturated fatty acids are found mainly in vegetable and nut oils, such as olive, peanut, and canola oil. They reduce blood cholesterol while not having the side effect of lowering high density lipids (HDL), the protective "good" cholesterol. Polyunsaturated fatty acids are found in certain fish and mainly in nuts and oils from plants, seeds, and soybeans. They reduce blood cholesterol, but an excess may lower high density lipids. When exposed to air, especially when heated, polyunsaturates undergo oxidation, making the oil rancid and producing trans fatty acids.

Vegetable shortenings and margarines have undergone a process called hydrogenation in which unsaturated oils are converted to a more solid form of fat. Hydrogenated oils act like saturated fats in the digestive process. This hardening of vegetable oils converts some of the naturally occurring fatty acids into trans fatty acids. The content of trans fatty acids generally increases to the extent an oil has been hydrogenated; for example, hard sticks of vegetable margarines may contain 25 to 35 percent of trans fats, whereas lightly hydrogenated oils (whipped or tub margarines) contain 5 percent or less. Trans fatty acids promote atherosclerosis. The metabolism of trans fatty acids produces free radicals. Free radicals can attack and penetrate a damaged cell and cause DNA changes, producing mutations. They are known to accelerate the aging process and can destroy healthy tissue. Butter, even with its high saturated fat, taken in small amounts, would be a better choice because it lacks trans fatty acids.

Cholesterol is a lipid or fat-related substance necessary for good health. It is a normal component of most body tissues, especially those of the brain, nervous system, liver, and blood. It is needed to form sex and adrenal hormones, vitamin D, and bile, which is necessary for the digestion of fats. Cholesterol deficiencies are unlikely, as the body manufactures most of what we need. If fats are eaten excessively, then cholesterol becomes stored throughout the body, particularly in the arteries. In the United States, the average fat consumption is 45 percent of daily caloric intake. The American Heart Association recommends that less than 30 percent of all daily calories come from fat. Many health experts go even further and recommend fat intake of 20 percent or even 10 percent to prevent common diseases such as cardiovascular disease and cancer. Saturated fat raises serum cholesterol in our bodies, and it is important to reduce the amount of fat we eat. In fact, saturated fats are more of a health problem than dietary cholesterol.

Fat is abundant in the following:

- fried foods (e.g., fried fish, chicken, and doughnuts)
- rich foods (e.g., premium ice cream and pastries)
- greasy foods (e.g., spare ribs and bacon)
- added fats and oils (e.g., butter, margarine, mayonnaise, oils)
- most snack foods (e.g., chips and cookies)

Fat can be hidden; that is, it may be buried in food where you neither see it nor expect to find so much of it. Muffins, hot dogs, and many crackers and sauces are surprisingly high in fat. To reduce the fat in your diet, you can choose simply prepared foods without rich sauces and gravies. Instead of fried food, you can eat foods that are baked, broiled, steamed, poached, or grilled. Keep in mind that one order of fast-food French fries has about twelve grams of fat, while one baked potato (unadorned) has under one gram.

Good Fats

Essential fatty acids (EFAs) are essential because your body cannot produce them; they must be consumed. They are necessary for the production of prostaglandins, which influence normal function of the cardiovascular, reproductive, immune, and central nervous systems. They also help regulate energy production and fat metabolism. They are known as the "fat burning" fats.

Omega-3 and omega-6 oils contain EFAs. Omega-3s are found in flaxseed, unrefined canola oil, cold water fish (salmon, mackerel, herring, or lake trout), wheat germ oil, walnuts, pumpkin seeds, and hemp seed oil. Omega-6s are in borage, evening primrose, unrefined corn, safflower, sunflower, and soybean oils. While there are numerous benefits from the intake of omega-3 and omega-6 oils, their absorption can be inhibited by stress, pollution, alcohol consumption, excess sugar intake, and trans fatty acids.

The main point to remember about fat intake is to limit your overall fat consumption to less than 30 percent of the total calories you consume each day. We believe 10 to 20 percent is best. Choose foods that contain unrefined monounsaturated fats like extra virgin olive oil or cold pressed canola oil. Include omega-3 and omega-6 fats. A greater proportion of omega-3 is important. Avoid making up for a reduced fat intake by eating high caloric "nonfat" foods.

Including a balance of fats may improve overall metabolism while maintaining that "full feeling" obtained from a typical American high-fat diet.

More About Cholesterol

Elevated cholesterol is one of the major risk factors for heart disease. The National Cholesterol Education Program suggests that everyone over the age of twenty have a cholesterol test, especially if there is a family history of heart problems, stroke, or other circulatory ailments. Testing for just the total cholesterol is incomplete. It is important to know your high density lipid, or HDL ("good"), and low density lipid, or LDL ("bad"), cholesterol levels. The more HDL the better. In a sense, the HDL acts to knock off the sticky LDL that clogs the arteries. It's desirable to have total cholesterol below 200, the LDL below 130 and the HDL above 45 for men and 55 for women. Some sources even recommend HDL to be above 60.

Thirty minutes of aerobic exercise three or four times a week may be all you need to raise the level of beneficial HDL in your bloodstream. Also, if you're a smoker, stopping can raise your HDL.

Following a low-fat, low cholesterol diet can usually reduce your blood cholesterol by about 15 percent, thus lowering your risk of heart disease by 30 percent. Individual results will vary, depending on genetic makeup and former eating habits.

Proteins

Next to water, protein is the most plentiful substance in the body (18 percent to 20 percent by weight). Protein is one of the most important elements for the maintenance of good health and vitality and is of primary importance in the growth and development of all body tissues. When it comes to energy, proteins are slow to digest and thus may be likened to efficient hardwoods, which create a slow-burning but steady fire. Every naturally occurring food contains some protein, so the sources are indeed abundant.

Twenty-two different amino acids are required to build all the proteins humans need. Fourteen of these can be manufactured within the body. The other eight cannot be easily synthesized by the body and must be supplied in the diet with regularity and in proper proportion. These eight are known as essential amino acids. If just one essential amino acid is missing, even temporarily, protein synthesis will fall to a very low level or stop altogether. The result is that all amino acids are reduced in the same proportion as the amino acid that is low or missing. To use another analogy with regard to protein utilization, proteins are like words, and the amino acids that comprise them are like letters. When protein is digested, it is taken apart and the letters are made available to spell whatever new words the body needs. In order to spell all the words necessary, a good supply of all the letters of the alphabet is imperative.

Foods containing protein may or may not contain all the essential amino acids. When a food contains all the essential amino acids, it is termed a "complete protein." Foods that lack or are extremely low in any one of the essential amino acids are called "incomplete proteins." Most meats and dairy products are complete protein foods, while most vegetables and fruits are incomplete protein foods. To obtain a complete protein meal from incomplete proteins, one must combine foods carefully so that those weak in an essential amino acid will be balanced by those adequate in the same amino acid.

The Function of Amino Acids

Amino acids are the chemical units or the "building blocks," as they are popularly called, that make up proteins. Protein could not exist without the proper combination of amino acids. In the human body, protein substances make up the muscles, ligaments, tendons, organs, glands, nails, hair, and body fluids (except for bile and urine). Proteins are essential for the growth of bones. Enzymes, hormones, and genes are also made up of various proteins. The central nervous system cannot function without amino acids, which act as neurotransmitters or as precursors to the neurotransmitters. They are necessary in order for the brain to receive and send messages. In addition to their other vital functions, amino acids enable vitamins and minerals to perform their jobs properly. Even if the vitamins and minerals are absorbed and assimilated rapidly, they will not be effective unless amino acids are present.

Complete proteins are necessary for sustenance of life. The following food combinations add up to a complete protein. By adding any of the following combinations to meals, the body will not require animal protein. Strict vegetarians must remember that they require vitamin B_{12} supplementation, as this vitamin is found almost exclusively in meat.

Beans form a complete protein when combined with one of the following foods:	Brown rice forms a complete protein when combined with one of the following foods:
Cheese	Beans
Nuts (all)	Nuts
Sesame seeds	Wheat
Wheat	Cheese
Corn	Sesame seeds
Rice	
Seeds (all)	

All soybean products, such as tofu and soy milk, are complete proteins. Cornmeal fortified with L-lysine makes a complete protein. A combination of any grain, all nuts, seeds, legumes, and a variety of mixed vegetables also makes a complete protein.

Minerals and Vitamins

Minerals are naturally occurring elements found in the earth. From the mineral salts contained in rocks and through the long process of erosion and soil formation, minerals make their way from the soil to plants and herbivorous animals. They function as coenzymes, which facilitate absorption, enabling the body to quickly and accurately perform its activities. They are needed for the proper composition of body fluids, the formation of blood and bone, and the maintenance of healthy nerve function.

Minerals belong to two groups: (1) macro (bulk) minerals and (2) micro (trace) minerals. Bulk minerals include calcium, magnesium, sodium, potassium, and phosphorus. The body needs these in larger amounts than trace minerals. Trace minerals include zinc, iron, copper, manganese, chromium, selenium, and iodine. Although only minute quantities of trace minerals are needed, they are important for good health. Because minerals are stored primarily in the body's bone and muscle tissue, it is possible to overdose on minerals if an extremely large dose is taken. However, toxic amounts will accumulate only if massive amounts are taken for a prolonged period of time.

Some mineral supplements are available in chelated form, which means that the minerals are attached to a protein molecule that transports them to the bloodstream to enhance absorption. Once a mineral is absorbed, it is carried by the blood to the cells and then transported across the cell membrane in a form that can be utilized by the cell. After the mineral enters the body, it competes with other minerals for absorption; therefore minerals should be taken in balanced amounts. For example, too much zinc can deplete the body of copper. Excessive calcium intake can affect magnesium absorption.

Vitamins, like minerals, function as coenzymes. They are not sources of energy, but they do determine and direct the ways in which ingested foods are assimilated and distributed. Vitamins are not components of major body structures but aid in the building of these structures.

All natural vitamins are organic food substances found only in living things (i.e., plants and animals). There are about twenty substances that are believed to be active as vitamins in human nutrition. Each of these vitamins is present in varying quantities in specific foods and each is absolutely necessary for proper growth and maintenance of health. With a few exceptions, the body cannot synthesize vitamins; they must be supplied in the diet or in dietary supplements.

Vitamins are usually distinguished as being water-soluble or fat-soluble. The water-soluble vitamins—B-complex, C, and the compounds termed "bioflavonoids"—are usually measured in milligrams. The fat-soluble vitamins—

A, D, E, and K—are measured in units of activity known as International Units (IU) or United States Pharmacopoeia Units (USP).

Nutritionists believe that fat-soluble vitamins are best absorbed if taken before meals, while water-soluble ones should be taken between or after meals.

Functional Foods

There is no current generally accepted definition for functional foods. One universally accepted opinion is that they are profitable for food manufacturers. Market projections predict double-digit growth for the next ten to thirty years. Functional foods are said to provide a physiological benefit beyond basic nutrition. For instance, we are now seeing corn chips with echinacea, an herbal immune system booster, or herbal teas with various boosters.

Functional foods have existed to a very small degree since the 1920s, when iodine was added to salt to prevent goiter. Then vitamin D was added to milk to boost calcium uptake, and flour became enriched with various vitamins. In recent years, there has been a flood of newly fortified foods on the market. In 1993, the FDA began approving health claims, such as "a diet low in saturated fat and cholesterol can reduce the risk of heart disease," on the labels of approved foods. So far, the FDA has approved roughly ten health claims. To skirt the approval process, food manufacturers have stepped up their "structure or function" claims (i.e., the food or additive can affect the structure or function of the body). So, if a food is not healthy enough to meet the FDA criteria for health claims, the manufacturer may make its own claim, such as "promotes a healthy heart."

Naturally occurring whole foods have a large variety of nutrients that act synergistically. That is to say, if one nutrient is missing, some of the other nutrients may not be available to benefit the body. Many commercially available functional foods emphasize only a few nutrients to the exclusion of others, thus creating an imbalance. Furthermore, the Foundation of Innovation in Medicine reports that "ninety-five percent of functional foods have not been clinically tested and are making claims unsupported by clinical data." At the same time, the American Dietetics Association (ADA) position statement on functional foods states, "The amounts of naturally occurring components contained in foods, in portions commonly consumed, may be inadequate to achieve optimal health benefits. The enhancement of foods may be a reasonable approach to achieving optimal health."

There's an inherent danger in leading the public to believe that one can compensate for an inadequate diet by eating fortified corn chips or consuming vitamin enhanced fruit drinks. Nature's functional foods, fruits, vegetables, whole grains, and legumes, are loaded with nutrients or phytochemicals that may cut the risk of cancer, heart disease, high blood pressure, eye disease, and other health problems. A balance of whole foods still provides the best choice for optimal nutrition. Whole foods have an added benefit in that they don't need to support a large advertising budget, so they're much less costly.

*You don't have to cook fancy or complicated masterpieces—
just good food from fresh ingredients.*

—Julia Child

Simple Suggestions for Healthy Eating

- Begin early. Those who eat a healthy breakfast generally feel less hungry throughout the day.
- Avoid fried or sauteed foods. Choose baked, steamed, poached, broiled, or roasted options.
- Eat smaller amounts more frequently rather than two or three large meals.
- Add variety by eating different foods each day.
- Use small amounts of meat for flavoring, if you eat it at all. Trim the fat from red meats and remove skin from chicken.
- Eat slowly. It takes about fifteen minutes for your brain to register that you are full. Put the fork down between bites. Eat only while sitting, not while driving or on the run.
- Eat at least five servings a day of fresh fruits or vegetables.
- Choose breads with whole grains, not just "wheat," but "whole wheat."
- Choose foods low in fat and sugar and high in complex carbohydrates and fiber (i.e., whole grains, beans, pasta, fruits, and vegetables).
- "Drink water as your beverage of choice. [It is] the only drink for a wise man." (Henry David Thoreau)
- Incorporate foods that are labeled and certified organic. These are foods that have not been treated with pesticides.

Water, Water Everywhere

The need for water in the human body is absolutely critical. The average amount of water in the human body is about 60 percent of total body weight. We rely upon water for digestion, cooling the body, elimination, and, of course, circulation of nutrients to every cell in the body. Failure to replenish the supply will mean death. Quite literally, you have to drink to live. The need for water is clear!

Nutritional Considerations • 19

The exact amounts of water required daily will vary depending upon the foods you eat, the temperature and humidity of the air, your amount of exercise, and your individual rate of metabolism. (Some of us just sweat more than others.) A general rule of thumb is to drink the amount in ounces equal to half your body weight. So, someone who weighs 120 pounds should drink at least 60 ounces (two quarts) of water daily. Fortunately, supplying this element is not a problem. We get water by drinking liquids and by eating solid foods, some of which are more than 90 percent water (e.g., carrots, lettuce, tomatoes, and watermelons). We also get water from body cells as a byproduct of metabolism. But the main source for replacement needs to come from drinking water. And the cleaner it is, the better.

Facts About Water Intake and Loss

Without air, life ceases in six to ten minutes. Without water, life ends in about 72 hours. Without eating, one could survive 30 to 40 days.

The average adult's body contains about eleven gallons of water. Without exercise, the average adult loses about three quarts per day through the kidneys, respiration, and perspiration. An additional quart is lost through 45 to 60 minutes of exercise per day or from living in a hot, humid climate. In about one hour of exercise, 1 to 2 percent of the body's water is lost. A loss of 5 percent results in dizziness, headaches, and aphasia (difficulty expressing oneself verbally). Death can result with a 15 to 20 percent loss (one-fifth of total volume).

Hydration depends on a balance between water added from external sources and water lost through urine, stools, expired air, and skin. Most of our daily water intake enters by the oral route, but a small amount is also synthesized in the body as a result of oxidation of hydrogen in food; this quantity ranges between five and eight ounces.

About half of our water intake is lost through urine, about 15 percent through sweat and feces, and about 35 percent through evaporation from the respiratory tract and by diffusion through the skin. Water lost through respiration and through the skin (without apparent sweating) constitutes "insensible loss," which is a volume of nearly one quart per day in a resting, healthy adult. Fever or sweating increases this loss. In very hot weather, additional water loss in the sweat occasionally rises to as much as one and a half quarts in an hour, which obviously can rapidly deplete the body fluids.

Exercise increases the loss of water in two ways. First, it increases the rate of respiration, which promotes increased water loss through the respiratory tract. Second, and much more important, exercise increases body heat and consequently is likely to result in more sweating.

Dehydration refers to water depletion. You can suspect dehydration might be present when there is a history of inadequate fluid intake, vomiting, diarrhea, or sweating. The main physical signs are decreased skin elasticity, postural hypotension (dizziness when changing positions), and, in more severe cases, lethargy, weakness, confusion, and drastically reduced urine output.

Fluid Replacement

Fluid replacement is a critical part of exercise in any season or climate. This is especially true for endurance sports, such as marathon running, long-distance cycling, or strenuous hiking, when you can easily lose a quart of water in an hour. In endurance activities, water loss can be severe, potentially producing heat exhaustion or heat stroke.

Overall, water is the best replacement fluid. Since the body loses water throughout the day, it is best to take it in gradually. Small portions of six to eight ounces are assimilated more easily than larger ones.

During the past ten years, some researchers have found that drinks containing up to 10 percent sugar are usually as well absorbed as water. Moreover, when consumed during a strenuous endurance event, sugared beverages may help the body conserve its carbohydrate stores, maintain normal blood sugar levels, and thus delay fatigue. Fruit juices and soft drinks contain more than 10 percent sugar, so they should be diluted. Specially formulated sports drinks such as Gatorade supply the optimal amount of carbohydrates (6 to 9 percent concentration) for endurance exercise. These sports drinks are nutritionally similar to diluted juice or soft drinks, only more expensive. Except under the most extreme circumstances, there is no need to replace electrolytes by consuming special drinks or mineral supplements—your normal diet will do the trick.

Caffeine is not a good ingredient for fluid replacement. Its stimulating properties may overwork an already overworked body. Also, caffeine is a potent diuretic, thus increasing fluid loss through urination. Carbonated beverages are thought to be appropriate as a fluid replacement option. However, the carbonation (which is carbon dioxide) is an unusable waste product that the body works hard to eliminate. Carbon dioxide also delays digestion by neutralizing stomach acids. Alcoholic beverages are poor fluid replacement choices, as they promote dehydration, hamper coordination, and impair athletic performance.

The most important thing is to drink—even if you don't feel thirsty! Thirst is satisfied long before you have replenished lost fluids. For optimal hydration during strenuous exercise, especially in hot weather, drink at least 16 to 20 ounces of fluid two hours before exercising and another eight ounces 15 minutes before. While exercising, sip four to six ounces every 15 to 20 minutes.

After exercising, drink enough to replace the fluid you've sweated off. You can weigh yourself before and after your workout; then drink 16 ounces for each pound lost.

Unfortunately, thirst isn't always a good indicator of the body's need for fluids. It's possible to lose two quarts of water before you notice your fluid loss by feeling thirsty. If, after prolonged exercise, you depend merely on your thirst, it can take several days to reestablish your body's fluid balance. So, go find a large glass, fill it with good clean water, and keep it near you all day long for sipping. And refill it when it's empty!

Chapter 3

Daily Awareness

The beginning of all disease processes starts with postural distortion.

—Hans Selye

As a society, we live life at breakneck speed. Some of us rush home from work to take the kids to after-school practice or lessons. Others work several jobs trying to make ends meet. Others create more and more *things* to do in their lives. (Where have we heard this before?) By the end of the day, most of us are fairly wiped out both mentally and physically. Our bodies hurt, and our minds are filled with noise from the day. We've forgotten how to just be quiet and enjoy a more leisurely life.

"What does this have to do with anything?" you ask. "I already know I'm catapulting through life and I can't do anything about it! I still have to . . ."

We'll tell you why. We've already described what you can do in the area of nutrition. Now we dedicate this chapter to information about how you can be more comfortable in your body both day and night, and we give you some examples to show how it can be done.

Our intent is to increase your awareness of how you use your body. We hope to encourage you to continually find new and improved ways to do the same old thing with much better results and less wear and tear on your body. Have fun!

"How?" you ask. "Posture," we say simply, "posture and body mechanics." Yep, two more things to remember, but they too will become habits. It can be quite a fun challenge to become more aware of your body each day and to discover new and better ways to accomplish the same tasks that once caused you discomfort.

We're going to plunge right into this now. Let's start with waking up in the morning.

Do you feel discomfort or pain in your low back when you wake up? Are you achy? Then tonight, put a pillow between your knees if you're sleeping on your side and another one under your neck to keep it in a neutral position.

Does your wrist bother you? Try to keep from curling your hand in a fist while you're sleeping. Sometimes snuggling with your loved one or hugging a pillow can help keep it straight.

Does a shoulder hurt when you lie on your side? Relieve the pressure by using another small pillow under the side of your ribs so that the shoulder is cradled between that one and the one under your neck. Or lie on your back with a pillow under your knees and another one under your neck. The key to remember here is to maintain a neutral position—that is, a position where your bones and joints are in line with each other, especially in the hip, back, and neck. It does take some time to become accustomed to all those pillows, but, given time, you will.

Okay, back to your achy body. This morning take a few more minutes and stay in bed. Then, slowly bring your knees to your chest and rock gently from side to side, feeling the circulation reenter your back as the ache slowly subsides.

Feel a little bit better now? Then it's time for that hot shower! While you're in the shower, feel the hot water beat down upon your neck, shoulders, and back. Feel the warmth relax those muscles; the tension is easing up.

Now slowly stretch your neck. Bring the right ear down to the right shoulder. Keep that shoulder down, you're trying to isolate and stretch just your neck! Feel the hot water continue to warm up the muscles as you do. Hold that stretch for two long seconds. That's one thousand one, one thousand two. And repeat that stretch four to ten times, depending on your fitness level. Do the same stretch on the left side. Now, standing erect and looking straight ahead, slowly turn your head and look over one shoulder. Feel the stretch for two seconds and return to start. Do this stretch four to ten times and repeat on the other side.

Start again for another stretch by standing erect and looking straight ahead. Then slowly tuck your chin to your neck and roll your head down. Feel the hot water warm your neck as you stretch. Hold the stretch for two seconds and repeat as before.

No pain is your gain! You need only stretch to light irritation. If the stretch hurts, then return to neutral and reposition yourself.

Continue stretching as you get ready for the day. For example, as you pull on your shirt, with your arm outstretched bring your hand up as if to say, "stop!" and repeat the action. Oh, it's going to be a fine day with a morning routine such as this.

Here's how some of our clients come into our office and what we tell them.

Martha comes in for a monthly massage. Her ongoing complaint is pain in both of her wrists, upper back, neck, and shoulders. Her doctor has diagnosed carpal tunnel syndrome. Martha is a middle school secretary. Her duties include typing, computer work, and frequent telephone use. In addition to all that, she also uses sign language because she works in the deaf department at her school. Recently, she has experienced difficulty while doing simple things around her home—putting the dishes away or even blow-drying her hair. All of these repetitive activities and sustained postures contribute to her symptoms.

Here are some suggestions we give Martha:

- Continue with her regular massages, since these give her some relief.
- Become aware of her posture during her work activities and consider how she can modify the posture, the activities, or both. Some modifications might be to make sure the typewriter is at a proper height for her, that the computer monitor and keyboard are adjusted correctly for her needs, and that she *not* cradle the telephone between her ear and shoulder. For long telephone conversations, Martha could consider using the opposite hand to ear, wearing a headset, or using a speakerphone. Her feet should be resting comfortably on the floor and she should sit in a chair that offers good support for her low back. If she is not able to obtain a new chair, then using cushions and props can help fit the chair to her individual needs. She should avoid leaning forward, lower her shoulders, keep breathing, and periodically (perhaps every thirty to sixty minutes) take short breaks of one to five minutes to stretch.
- Stretch frequently and properly—this is one of the keys to successful management of her symptoms. She can do stretches upon waking, in the shower, after dinner, or even at the movies.

The pain and discomfort that Martha experiences is, in large part, due to her job. There are numerous names that that are given to the conditions or syndromes like Martha's. You may have heard them referred to as cumulative trauma disorder, repetitive stress injury, or overuse syndrome. They are all similar. Lauren A. Hebert, in his book *The Neck Arm Hand Book,* defines cumulative trauma disorder as a "disease of the musculoskeletal system, produced by a gradual build-up of tiny amounts of damage that occur on a daily basis as a result of repetitive motion and/or sustained posture and is focused to a specific part of the body."

Technology has advanced to such a degree that we could very easily stay in one place all day long, moving only the same small muscle groups over and over again. The checkout person in the grocery store no longer has to pick up the can of beans to find the price and then turn to enter the amount in the cash register. He simply pushes the items across the scanner with little break in between. His head is bent forward, his shoulders are rounded, and I would just bet his feet really hurt. Is it any wonder that we are seeing so many checkout persons wearing wrist braces and back supports? The typist's job has also become automated. He is now a computer operator. Who of you out there is old enough to remember the days of the manual, nonelectric typewriter? The repetitive motion of typing was once broken up by the simple act of changing the paper or a ribbon. Those actions no longer exist. And walking across the room to look up words in the dictionary or the thesaurus is no longer necessary, since they are very conveniently right inside our computers, accessed by a simple touch of a button.

But think of it. Touching a button really isn't so simple when it is the primary action we perform most of the day, day after day. As we sit or stand in one place long enough, we begin to squirm. Our posture begins to suffer and consequently we become tired, our posture becomes even worse, and, boy, are we in trouble now! Addressing the fatigue may be key to addressing the problem of cumulative trauma disorder. And it is the responsibility of everyone in the workplace, both employee and employer, to address the problems of both poor work environment and poor work habits to combat the effects.

Cumulative trauma disorders are preventable. Sometimes the answer can be as simple as setting a timer or alarm clock to go off at a designated time, perhaps every 30 to 60 minutes. If the clock is placed on the other side of the room, that person will need to, at the very least, get up and turn it off. And during the time of that two-minute walk, that office worker can perform some very productive stretches that will help alleviate shoulder, neck, and arm tension, not to mention gain some very important circulation throughout the body. Don't have time, you say? Two to five minutes each hour is a very inexpensive way to prevent a $30,000+ operation for a cumulative trauma disorder.

Carpal tunnel syndrome is one of the more common repetitive stress injuries we hear about and can be the end result of long-term neck and shoulder tension. Repetitive motion is not the only culprit. Sustained posture can be as damaging if not more than repetitive motion. If someone is sitting for long periods of time without much movement, say while driving a truck across the country, tiny muscles are constantly contracting in the neck and shoulders to try and maintain that posture. It is very demanding and can consume huge amounts of energy without us realizing it. Not only that, but small blood vessels and nerves can be entrapped by the sustained contraction, limiting their circulatory effects to the arm. So in the long run, tissue repair is hampered by the loss of the nutrient/waste exchange by the blood vessels, and nerve irritability can occur, creating pain and numbness. These things can be prevented. They can be managed.

More and more companies are employing an ergonomics team to survey the job site and employee work postures to determine how to best adapt the work to the person, rather than forcing the person to adapt to the work. Ergonomics is the scientific study of human work. It takes into consideration the physical and mental capabilities and limitations of the employee and how he or she interacts with the tasks, methods, tools, equipment, and environment. In 1994, the Bureau of Labor Statistics Annual Occupational Injury/Illness Survey reported that 65 percent of time off work due to illness was because of cumulative trauma disorders.

The same principles of ergonomics at the worksite can also be applied to home and recreational activities. Weekend home and yard maintenance play significant roles in repetitive stress injuries. Now there are special rakes and shovels available to help maintain a neutral position in the wrist. They have angled handles that let the wrist joint remain straight and decrease your chance of injury. Believe it or not, there is even a correct way to vacuum. Instead of using the vacuum as an extension of your arm, hold it close to your hip and let it follow your feet as you walk back and forth. This will reduce the repetitive stress on the neck, shoulder, arm, and low back that results from a constant reaching method. As you complete your chores, think about these ideas and how you can continue to incorporate changes into your routine to increase your comfort level. And now that those chores are finished, let the games begin!

Scenario 1: Your daughter is in Little League and really needs some batting practice. As you get the bat and ball out of the closet, achy shoulder memories from the last season come to mind. How can you do things differently this year? Start off by getting into the habit of having both of you of warm up your muscles before you play. Then remember to take breaks from throwing the ball, stretch periodically, and drink water. Give yourself adequate time to cool down afterwards. If you still feel sore, use ice on that area.

Scenario 2: Your favorite hobby is needlepoint, but your neck is sore, your eyeglasses keep slipping, your wrist hurts, and your low back aches. What can you do? You want to finish the sampler in time for the baby shower. There are many changes you can make in this situation. First, get a good pair of glasses that stay put on your face and make sure the prescription is appropriate for the type of work you are doing. That adjustment alone will help your neck. Then be sure your chair is comfortable and gives you plenty of support. Lighting should be directly overhead; reposition it if there are shadows on your work area. Have you tried using a needlepoint stand so that both hands are free and you can use the double-hand method of stitching? If so, be sure it's at the correct height for you. Remember to keep your wrists in a neutral position—relaxed and straight. Keep both feet flat on the floor. Try pinching your shoulder blades together and pulling in your lower abdominal muscles from time to time to maintain a correct posture. Good luck with your deadline!

Scenario 3: You're a computer jockey! That's right, you qualify for the title of "industrial athlete." The proper chair is essential for you. It should support your low back and have adjustable arm rests so that your wrists are straight and forearms are parallel to the floor while using the keyboard and mouse. Your knees should be slightly lower than your hips, and your feet should be flat on the floor or on a foot rest. The monitor should be between eighteen and thirty inches away, and the top line of the screen should be just below eye level to keep the neck straight. Adjustable platforms can be used if workstations are shared. Documents should be positioned similarly and near the screen. You should be able to adjust the screen's brightness and contrast with ease. Prevent glare on the screen by placing your monitor between overhead lights and perpendicular to the windows. Your hands and wrists should be in a neutral position during keying, and you should be careful that the nerves are not compressed against sharp edges. Take breaks to stretch; avoid a sustained posture.

The bottom line? You are responsible for your well-being. Become more aware of what you are doing in each situation, wherever you are, and how it affects your body. How can you modify your posture, environment, methods, and equipment so that you are comfortable and less prone to fatigue and overuse syndromes? We've compiled some tips to help you.

Postural Awareness

General Principles

- Keep your body in a neutral position. Your joints should be naturally aligned and your muscles relaxed.
- Avoid fatigue by changing position often, stretching whenever possible, and breathing (many of us forget to breathe regularly when we are engrossed in an activity).
- Contract your lower abdominal muscles and pinch your shoulder blades together.
- Stay hydrated; drink water throughout the day.
- Smile and laugh often. This does wonders for your spirit and relaxes your muscles as well.

Sitting Posture

- Find a good, adjustable chair with proper support (e.g., lumbar support, arm rests, bolsters) specific to the activity you must perform.
- Keep your feet flat on the floor or use a foot rest.
- Keep frequently used items close at hand to avoid awkward twisting or reaching movements.

Standing Posture

- Use antifatigue mats or shoe inserts. (Note: it is important to be sure the type of mat is appropriate for your job and/or that your shoes fit correctly with the type of insoles that you use.)

- Install a foot rail or something similar. Elevating one foot four or five inches will round out the lower back (a neutral position) and decrease pressure on the vertebral discs.
- Change your position often to increase circulation to muscles and decrease fatigue and pain.

Lifting Posture

- Keep objects close to your center of gravity (usually your abdomen) while you lift.
- If the object is on or low to the ground, lift with your legs by bending your knees; that is, do not bend over from the waist to lift. Instead, kneel down or squat to pick up the object and maintain a straight back.
- Avoid making awkward twisting or turning movements. Turn by using your feet instead.
- Break up the load to make it lighter.
- Take the time to make several lighter trips rather than carrying one heavy load.
- Avoid repetitive lifting or reaching overhead; use a stepstool or stepladder (make sure they're stable). If you use the objects often, then find a place for them at waist height.

Factors That Can Contribute to Cumulative Trauma Disorders

- Physical stress can produce fatigue and injury.
- Emotional and/or mental stress contribute to general fatigue and can create a lack of focus on the task at hand.
- Asymmetrical body structure, such as having one arm immobilized in a cast for six weeks, can cause the noninjured arm to become overused. Or, if one leg is shorter than the other, this can create an imbalance in the pelvis. A heel lift may be needed.
- Chemical imbalances caused by poor nutrition or abuse of substances like alcohol (dehydrates the body and reduces the uptake of nutrition) and tobacco (robs the tissues of oxygen and decreases their ability to repair themselves) can inhibit the body's natural immunity to disease and injury.
- Diseases such as arthritis and diabetes can make the body more vulnerable to cumulative trauma.
- Hormonal shifts in women can cause a fluid buildup that further reduces circulation to stressed areas and increases inflammation.
- Poor posture, especially the common forward-head posture, is a major risk factor.

Muscle Pain

Why do you have muscle pain? There are a number of possible reasons, but the underlying problem is the lack of oxygen (ischemia) in the blood. If the blood flow is restricted from a tight muscle or spasm (like a kink in a garden hose), less oxygen will be available to the area. With less blood flow and less oxygen getting to the muscle, there's also a buildup of metabolic waste products that can't leave the muscle. These waste products contain acids that create even more irritation in the tissues. Massage, stretching, reducing stress, and aerobic exercise all help muscles relax, allowing more oxygen-rich blood flow into the tissues and flushing out waste products.

Aerobic activity is one of the best methods to increase the oxygen distribution throughout your body. The way the body uses oxygen as its energy source is through rhythmic and continuous movement, which includes activities like walking, cycling, and swimming.

A regular flexibility program is a great way to ease the muscle tightness from stress and tension. Stretching not only lengthens and loosens muscles, it can be a form of meditation.

There are numerous massage techniques that are designed to loosen tight, constricted muscles, relieve spasms, and alleviate tension. The tightness and tension limits the amount of oxygen available to the muscles. The less oxygen there is, the more pain is experienced.

Tips for Comfortable Travel

Ow! You just woke up from napping on the plane, and your neck hurts. You're stiff and generally uncomfortable. The narrow seat and limited leg room make it difficult to position your low back comfortably. What's an air traveler to do? This section will address a few things you can do while on a plane or other modes of transportation; but that's only one part of the equation. In our Western culture, most view health as the absence of disease. Hippocrates said, "A wise man should consider that health is the greatest of human blessings." We view health as a form of wellness—a way of living more fully through behavior that allows us to feel good more often.

Travel Nutrition

Naturally, proper nutrition means that all the essential nutrients, carbohydrates, fats, protein, vitamins, minerals, and water are supplied and utilized in adequate balance to maintain optimal health and well-being. When traveling, it's even more important to increase your water and fiber intake, reduce fat intake, and get plenty of sleep. Eating healthfully does not mean feeling deprived. Healthful and delicious foods are abundant. Flexibility around exploring new tastes, textures, and traditions is the fun and creative part of making conscious, healthy choices.

Our bodies dehydrate quickly in the dry climate of an airplane or in the air conditioning of an automobile. Overall, water is the best replacement fluid; the worst are those that contain caffeine, carbonation, or alcohol. Caffeine (found in coffee, teas, and some sodas) is a potent diuretic, which increases fluid loss through urination. Carbonated beverages (sodas, mineral waters) are also not appropriate as a fluid replacement option because carbonation (carbon dioxide) is an unusable waste product that the body works hard to eliminate. Carbon dioxide also delays digestion by neutralizing stomach acids. Alcoholic beverages are poor fluid replacement choices, as alcohol promotes dehydration. The best thing you can do while traveling is drink plenty of water.

Since travel has become such a common way of life in our increasingly mobile society, we offer the following example to illustrate the point of this discussion.

You rush to pack and arrive at the airport on time, all the while lugging heavy bags to the gate and fighting the crowds. You finally have a chance to relax once you're on the plane. You sit down and realize your body just doesn't conform to the seat design. What to do?

- Use pillows and blankets as rolls and cushions to support your low back and neck. There are also many products on the market for lumbar and neck support that are easy to carry.
- Prop your feet up on your flight bag to help take pressure off the backs of your legs.
- Change positions often.
- Lean forward, propping your elbows on the tray table and your forehead in your hands.
- Alternate pulling one knee at a time up to your chest.
- Change the position of the seat.
- Walk/stand for short periods.
- Practice relaxation techniques through rhythmic, slow, deep breathing. Your body naturally relaxes on the exhale.
- Do stretching and isometric exercises while in your seat: slightly tilting pelvis, hiking hips, shrugging shoulders, pinching shoulder blades together, contracting and relaxing buttocks, contracting and relaxing feet and calves.
- Roll a golf ball, handball, or wooden foot massager under your feet to stimulate circulation and promote relaxation.

Chapter 4

Specific Health
Problems

The conditions described in this chapter are perhaps the most common and most annoying musculoskeletal conditions experienced by a vast number of people. We have synthesized the most salient points of various conditions into clearly understandable terms. With each condition, there is a section that describes its origins and how it evolves into a problem, what aggravates it, and what you can do to minimize its effects. Suggestions for self-management and stretches are listed so you can gain control over the condition rather than allow it to control you.

This information is not meant to diagnose or replace appropriate medical care. Our intent is to empower you with important information that can augment medical care and even prevent more serious complications. This information may also be useful as a starting point for asking questions of your health care provider. Fear and ignorance are counterproductive. The more you know and understand about the many facets of your health (or ill health) and the more you can focus on your abilities, the more able you become to move beyond the restrictive boundaries of your aches and pains.

Arthritis

What Is It?

Arthritis is not a single disease. It is an umbrella term for over 100 different rheumatic diseases, syndromes, and conditions that affect the joints or the supportive tissues surrounding them. The most common types of arthritis are osteoarthritis and rheumatoid arthritis, with osteoarthritis being the more prevalent and milder of the two.

Rheumatoid arthritis (RA) is an autoimmune disease, which means the immune system malfunctions and attacks the body's own tissue. It's an inflammatory process that creates swelling in the synovial membrane or joint lining and affects over seven million Americans. The swelling and pain are present in several joints and chiefly present in the small joints of the hands, wrists, elbows, shoulders, feet, ankles, and knees. It is usually bilateral; that is, it affects both sides of the body at the same time. Besides swelling, RA symptoms include redness around the joint, warmth, pain, tenderness, stiffness, nodules, fatigue, muscle aches, and fever. Heredity plays a role in contracting RA. The onset can be triggered by an infection in a genetically susceptible person. It may appear in children approaching adolescence or in adults in their twenties to fifties. Seventy-five percent of individuals affected are female. Approximately 0.5 percent of the U.S. population is affected. Rheumatoid arthritis is more painful than other forms of arthritis and can cause deformities in its advanced stages.

Treatment for RA is typically aggressive pharmaceutical intervention, such as experimental immunostimulants, systemic corticosteroids, chemotherapeutic agents, and analgesics. Joint replacement surgery is an option in severe instances of joint deterioration. Type of disease and disease severity should be key factors in the decision for surgery. Replacement of the larger joints, such as the hip, knee, and shoulder, is generally very effective in eliminating pain, reducing deformity, and restoring function. Surgical replacement of the smaller joints, such as the elbow, wrist, and ankle, has been largely unsuccessful.

Osteoarthritis (OA) is a condition of overuse and wear and tear of the joints that affects about sixteen million Americans. It is not related to immune system problems. Osteoarthritis involves chemical and structural changes in cartilage as well as hardening of the bone and formation of bone spurs around the joints that ultimately restricts mobility. Typically, OA involves only a few joints (the ones most overused) and may only be on one side of the body, unlike the bilateral nature of RA. Osteoarthritis develops slowly and manifests itself through symptoms of pain and stiffness. It develops most commonly in the weight-bearing joints such as the knees, hips, and spine. Severity of symptoms varies between individuals. Unfortunately, with increasing age and repetitive patterns, many of us will have some symptoms of arthritis creep into our existence.

Conventional medical approaches for the treatment of OA center around medication for pain relief and nonsteroidal antiinflammatory drugs (NSAIDs). A good way to determine the desirability of any arthritis treatment is to ask whether it is active or passive. Active therapies like exercise, visualization, or stress management methods require you to take an active role in your own health maintenance by using your muscles or your mind. We believe active therapies are much more successful than passive therapies, which have you swallow a pill or have something done to you by someone else while you do nothing. The more you know about your condition, the more control you can have over it and the less frightening and mysterious it becomes. A Stanford University study of 224 arthritis patients bears this out. It found that educating arthritis patients about their disorder was as effective in reducing pain as any of the most popular arthritis medications.

While medications may be necessary in the treatment of arthritis, the most important thing you can do to help yourself is to exercise. Rhythmic activities, such as cycling, walking, swimming (or water exercises), and stretching, reduce stiffness and aid in joint lubrication, as well as increase the release of endorphins. These are natural morphinelike opiates that switch off pain by binding to pain receptors in the brain. As a result, depression and anxiety are decreased due to the increased levels of comfort in the body. The good news is that most people with arthritis are able to exercise.

What Aggravates It?

Lack of activity and being overweight are perhaps the greatest factors that aggravate osteoarthritis or rheumatoid arthritis. Because movement creates pain, many arthritis patients quit moving. Lack of movement creates more stiffness and thus more pain. So, it is most important to gradually build up your exercise tolerance in order to move with less pain. Application of moist heat may be necessary before exercise in some instances.

The stress of bearing excessive weight softens and frays the cartilage that pads the ends of bones in a joint. The cartilage wears thin, hardens, becomes pitted, and can no longer absorb shock within the joint. There is well-documented evidence that suggests that being overweight and having a sedentary lifestyle are primary precipitators in the development of OA. A Johns Hopkins School of Medicine study found that men in their twenties who are twenty pounds or more overweight almost double their risk of developing OA in the knees and hips in later life. Osteoarthritis is seldom observed in any active person who stays fit and trim.

Other factors that aggravate the symptoms of arthritis are stress and feelings of hopelessness and helplessness. Hope is good medicine for arthritis patients. Hope allows you to see arthritis as a challenge to overcome. It instills a sense of control and self-advocacy. Stress occurs when one must adjust to a change or life event that is perceived as threatening or hostile to comfort, safety, or well-being. Emotions of anger, hostility, fear, and resentment all create stress. Enduring an unwanted disease can certainly produce any or all of these emotions. The resulting stress tightens muscles and keeps the body in a state of heightened alert, a "fight or flight" mode. In this mode, the body cannot adequately rest, restore, and repair. Stress also impacts the immune system. With stress, immunity is suppressed, and the body is not able to fend off disease and RA flare-ups.

Conventional medical "wisdom" states that diet has no influence on arthritis. Well into the 1980s conventional medical wisdom also maintained that diet had no effect on heart disease. Now there is absolutely no doubt about the link between diet and cardiovascular health. Many studies on arthritis indicate that diet indeed can aggravate arthritic symptoms. A diet that contains red meat, high fats, sugar, and wine is known to aggravate symptoms. Studies also suggest that nightshade vegetables (tomatoes, peppers, etc.) can create more discomfort. Some physicians go as far as saying that following a vegan diet that restricts all animal products is a powerful pain reducer for RA.

Self-Help Measures

Moderate activity, activity, activity. About the only time activity should be restricted is when there is an acute flare-up. An exercise program should be regular and balanced between gentle strength training, aerobic fitness, and flexibility.

Energy Conservation

Principles of wise energy conservation need to be considered. That is, avoid exercises that produce excessive pain and fatigue.

- Several short periods of exercise throughout the day are of greater value than long periods of exercise. You may expect some discomfort while exercising, but stop if pain occurs.
- Plan to alternate work and rest periods.
- It's important to realize that you don't have to finish a task before you rest.

A key to living a full life is to learn your limitations and work within them. Strive for a balance between work, rest, and leisure activities.

Joint Protection

Do all you can to protect your joints from overuse or improper use.

- Avoid deforming postures, such as slouching or limb flexion.
- Choose a chair that gives proper support. Keep your head up, hips and shoulders against the chair back, and feet flat on the floor.
- Sit to work when you can.
- Invest in long-handled tools to avoid unnecessary bending and stretching.
- Try not to subject your joints to excessive weight.
- When moving heavy objects, use two hands to push instead of lifting or pulling.

- Use a larger joint in preference over a smaller one (i.e., carry a handbag strap over your shoulder instead of with your fingers).
- Avoid ulnar deviation (fingers slanting toward the little-finger side of the hand).
- To save wear and tear on your joints, use labor saving devices, such as an electric can opener, electric knife and mixer, or broad handled kitchen utensils.

Other Self-Help Measures

- Make efforts to lose weight if you are overweight.
- If certain joint movements are too painful, try moist heat to the area prior to exercise.
- Practice moving meditation such as tai chi, chi gong, or yoga.

Massage therapy, acupuncture, and certain herbs can be very beneficial. Certain nutrients are likely to be deficient in people with arthritis. Specific ones worth considering for supplementation include vitamins B-complex, C, D, and E, as well as calcium and magnesium.

Stretching Recommendations

Throughout the week, stretch the different regions of the body to ultimately stretch the entire body. Stretch the areas most affected by joint pain and strain several times a week. Try implementing at least two seven-minute routines a day.

Fibromyalgia and Chronic Fatigue Syndromes

What Is It?

Fibromyalgia Syndrome (FMS) is a condition of the muscles that manifests as pain throughout much of the body. The word *fibromyalgia* literally means pain of the muscle fibers (*algia* means pain; *fibromy* means muscle fibers). It is not a progressive disease. It does not put people in wheelchairs. It is a condition, with no known cause, that cycles between tolerable and severe in its symptoms. Many people with fibromyalgia say they ache all over. Their muscles feel like they've been overworked. The symptoms and onset of fibromyalgia are very similar to those of chronic fatigue syndrome (CFS), so close that researchers have classified FMS and CFS as one and the same. Fibromyalgia syndrome has a fatigue component but is largely a painful condition. Chronic fatigue syndrome has a pain component but is largely a condition of fatigue.

The onset of FMS/CFS seems to appear after a particularly severe viral/bacterial illness or after physical or emotional trauma. More women than men are afflicted. FMS/CFS can be present in people of all ages. Much of the current research as to the cause is centered around alterations in the neurotransmitter serotonin. Immune function, sleep physiology, and hormonal imbalances are also being studied. In our observations of people with FMS/CFS we wonder if onset could be related to "burning out the adrenals." The adrenal glands are overworked when the body is stressed. Illness, trauma, and psychological concerns all stress the body. When you couple a particularly difficult time in one's life with intense omnipresent daily stressors, it seems that the body's way of saying it needs a break is to totally "shut down" in order to get the rest it needs. The pain, fatigue, and other symptoms associated with FMS/CFS definitely command one's attention and force rest.

Those with FMS/CFS endure a variety of unpleasant symptoms that limit previously normal activities. The pain of fibromyalgia syndrome may be described as deep muscular aching, burning, throbbing, shooting, or stabbing. The fatigue experienced by those with FMS/CFS may range from mild tiredness to feeling totally drained of energy and having frequent "brain fog." Sleeping patterns are generally disturbed so that one awakens often through the night and feels unrefreshed and in pain in the morning. At least half of those with FMS/CFS report symptoms of irritable bowel syndrome, which presents as constipation, diarrhea, abdominal pain, and/or gas. Many people also report frequent headaches, tension, or migraines.

What Aggravates It?

Repetitive activities and physical overexertion are the most common things that limit relatively normal functioning. Changes in weather, particularly changes in barometric pressure, cold or drafty environments, hormonal fluctuations, stress, anxiety, or depression all contribute to symptom flare-ups.

Self-Help Measures

A common personality of those with FMS/CFS is an ambitious, active, responsible, "go getter" type. The greatest challenge is to harness the desire of doing things the way "I always used to do" and practice very conscious energy conservation. There are good days and bad days. Often when one has a good day, the tendency is to try to accomplish everything that has been delayed due to the previous bad days. This is when you can get into trouble and end up in bed for the next few days.

Conscious energy conservation means that when you are having a good day, keep it a good day. Whatever task you have, break it up into 15-minute segments and rest after each segment to assess if you really have enough energy to continue. Avoid repetitive motion. Certain days, the simple act of unloading a dishwasher may be too repetitive.

Become aware of how you use your body. Are you bending and reaching too much? Do your best to sit and stand in an erect posture and avoid slouching. Vacuuming is very strenuous work, especially with all the arm and shoulder movement. Try holding the vacuum near your hip and use your legs by walking forward and back instead of pushing the vacuum with your arms.

Many people benefit from regular therapeutic massage, and others do well with medication. Still others need both. Whatever the case, an understanding physician should manage overall care. Rheumatologists are the specialists who best understand FMS/CFS and who are probably most up to date on the latest research or treatment options.

Regular and mild aerobic exercise can keep the muscles in a more resilient condition by pumping more oxygen to all the tissues. This aids in fewer and less severe "bad days." This will also aid in better sleep-wake patterns. Of course, improving flexibility allows the muscles to relax more. It also lengthens the muscle fibers so there may be fewer knots in the muscles.

Stretching Recommendations

In the interest of energy conservation, do one to three of the seven minute routines throughout the day. Focus on the body areas where you experience the most discomfort. Attempt to stretch all regions of the body at least once a week.

Headache

What Is It?

Headaches are commonly categorized as tension, migraine, or sinus in origin. They may also be caused by a pathological disease process that is far less common than the other three causes.

Tension headaches are typically caused by physical or emotional stress. This includes factors such as eye strain, poor posture, a neck injury like whiplash, or even conditions such as temporomandibular joint dysfunction. The pain of a tension headache may feel like a hat is being worn too tight.

Migraine headaches are vascular in origin and are characterized by a preceding bout of bizarre sensory disturbances called auras. These may appear as a flashing wheel of lights. The pain often affects one side of the head and may be accompanied by nausea. There are numerous reasons for the blood vessels inside the head to become engorged with blood, and it is difficult to pinpoint the exact cause. Approximately 11 percent of the U.S. population experience migraines, and women are affected more often than men.

Sinus headaches arise from increased pressure in the sinus cavities in the area of the nose and eyes. Pressure in the nose, cheek, forehead, or temple areas may result from a sinus infection or allergies.

What Aggravates It?

Tension headaches are the most common type of headaches. Quite simply, tightness in the neck and shoulder muscles seems to be the most direct cause. In our experience, myofascial trigger points in any of the muscles of the neck and shoulders can "trigger" pain in the head, behind the eyes, at the base of the skull, and in the back or side of the head, or they can create that "tight band" feeling around the head. Deactivating these trigger points and relieving tension in the muscles through therapeutic massage often can decrease the frequency and intensity of tension headaches.

Certain foods are considered to initiate headaches in some people. These foods include nitrates (added to hot dogs, bacon, lunch meats, etc.), some sugar substitutes, and, heaven forbid, chocolate. Certain interactions between medications may cause headaches. Lack of appropriate fluid intake or too much fluid loss from sweating or diarrhea can bring on a headache. Avoid skipping meals to keep blood sugar at appropriate levels so the brain isn't stressed any further. Smoking and alcohol intake also increase the likelihood for headache development.

Posture at work or during leisure activities may aggravate the tension in the neck and shoulder muscles. Good lumbar support encourages the body to be more erect, thus lessening the tension in the neck and shoulder area. The classic way a headache may develop in relation to posture follows this pattern: Persistent leaning forward at a desk creates an imbalance and tension in the neck and shoulder region. These muscles become tight and grow less resilient. Add some time deadlines to your workload or couple this with some workplace conflict, and the muscles tighten even further. This often creates trigger points, which are areas in the muscle that have become very irritable. This irritability in the muscle spills over into nearby organs or muscle tissue and produces pain and causes the area to have more dysfunction, thus turning into a headache.

Since migraines are vascular, they don't necessarily follow the pattern of tension headache development. Migraines can be triggered by diet, weather, exercise, light, altitude, hormonal shifts, and emotions. Where migraines overlap with tension headaches is that tension in the neck and shoulder muscles can allow a migraine to be triggered more readily or make it more severe. Since the brain becomes engorged with blood during a migraine, the blood needs somewhere to go to bring relief. If there's a general state of tension in the muscles in the area, the ability for blood to circulate freely will be greatly diminished. Thus the pressure remains fairly high within the skull.

Self-Help Measures

The most obvious yet most difficult measure to incorporate to decrease or eliminate headaches is to slow down and have regular periods of rest and relaxation. The advertisements say, "for a normal everyday headache, take this medication, it's safe." Having a headache is not normal and should not be occurring every day or even every week. No medication is completely safe. Aspirin and ibuprofen, while effective for decreasing pain, fever, and inflammation, create gastrointestinal disturbances and may cause internal bleeding. Acetaminophen (Tylenol) does not have the stomach and intestinal side effects and is effective for decreasing pain and fever. It is, however, very toxic to the liver. An overdose with as few as thirty tablets can cause liver failure and death.

Tension headaches can be decreased or eliminated through a number of methods:

- engaging in regular and moderate exercise
- performing regular meditation
- reducing caffeine intake
- eating more whole foods and fewer fast or processed foods
- sitting quietly to eat meals, avoiding eating on the run
- increasing flexibility in the neck and shoulder muscles
- stopping smoking and tobacco use
- improving workplace ergonomics
- having regular sleep-wake patterns
- taking time for relaxation, hobbies, and varied recreational activities
- receiving periodic therapeutic massage or bodywork
- developing a trusting emotional support system with friends, family, and/or a therapist

Oftentimes a headache can be relieved by stopping a few minutes, slowing and deepening your breath, and visualizing a loosening of the muscles of the head and neck and by gently massaging your temples. Applying pressure to the origins of each eyebrow and to the webs on each hand between your thumb and index finger can also help relieve headache pain.

An effective self-help remedy for migraines requires a small bit of preparation but is well worth the minimal effort. At any point in the process of a migraine (earlier is better than later), lie on your back in a dark, quiet room. Place an ice pack under your neck, and place your feet in very warm water.

This creates a hydrostatic effect that pulls the blood from the head to the lower extremities. This remedy was widely used with great success before the dawning of the pharmaceutical age. The ice also interrupts the pain-spasm-pain cycle that may be simultaneously occurring in the neck muscles, and thus relaxes those tissues. The self-help measures listed for tension headaches are also quite helpful to reduce the occurrence and frequency of migraines.

Sinus headaches may need the assistance of medications like antihistamines or decongestants. Frequently in our practices of massage therapy, we find trigger points on the base of the skull that refer pain to the sinus area. Some individuals have noticed a reduction of "sinus attacks" after this treatment is administered. It is difficult to assess whether the sinus problem caused tension in the muscles and fascia of the head and neck, or if the muscles became so irritable that this irritability spilled over into nearby tissues. It's worth investigating if it means the possibility of reducing the intake of medication.

Stretching Recommendations

Doing the seven-minute neck and shoulder routines daily can create considerable relaxation and flexibility in the neck muscles, thereby reducing the frequency, duration, and intensity of headaches.

Temporomandibular Joint Dysfunction

What Is It?

Commonly referred to as TMJ, temporomandibular joint dysfunction (TMD) is a condition of pain or improper opening or movement of the jaw. Also known as myofascial pain dysfunction, TMD affects approximately 20 percent of all Americans. It is characterized by pain, clicking, popping, or uneven tracking with jaw movement. Dysfunction of the temporomandibular joint can refer pain to the neck, ears, and head.

There are three distinct views among physicians as to the origin of TMD. Some view it as mainly a muscular problem, whereby the muscles that attach to the jaw are too tight and cause accelerated wear and tear within the jaw joint. Many dentists view it as a disturbance in occlusal mechanics. That is, how the teeth meet and how chewing occurs may contribute to unusual forces within the joint. Still others regard TMD as a physical response to stress or psychological difficulties. The common component in all these views is that abnormal habitual movements of the jaw cause TMD.

What Aggravates It?

The jaw is designed to chew approximately five hundred times per day. As in other muscles and joints, overuse can create problems. Clenching the teeth or nighttime grinding of the teeth are common habits that overuse the jaw. Chewing gum or biting hard candy and nuts also places undue stress on the jaw. Other activities, such as playing the violin or a wind instrument, can place the jaw in positions that strain the muscles around the joint, ultimately causing jaw movement problems. Certain postural patterns, like a forward-head posture, create more compression within the joint and subsequently cause uneven wearing of the joint lining.

Self-Help Measures

Here are some tips for preventing or alleviating TMD:

- Increase postural consciousness by sitting erect and avoiding constantly leaning forward.
- Do not eat hard candies, nuts, and other overly crunchy foods.
- Do not chew ice.
- Try to breathe through your nose with your mouth closed.
- Become aware of sleeping positions that may push on one side of the jaw.
- Take frequent breaks from playing musical instruments, like the violin or wind instruments, as these tend to push the jaw into unusual positions.
- Stop chewing gum.
- Avoid the nervous habit of chewing on pencils or other hard objects.
- Use moist heat packs in the area of the temporomandibular joint.
- Massage your face, particularly along the jaw and in front of your ears.
- Massage the temple area and the sides of your head.

Stretching Recommendations

1. Sit in an erect position, place two fingers in your mouth behind the lower teeth and pull the jaw forward and then down. Hold for two seconds and release. Repeat six to ten times.

2. With a facial look of surprise, raise your eyebrows and open your mouth as wide as possible, to light irritation. Hold two seconds and release. Repeat six to ten times.

3. The seven-minute neck and shoulder routines will bring relief to the muscles related to the jaw.

Neck Pain

What Is It?

A frequent complaint, neck pain can result for a variety of reasons. It can be acute or chronic. The neck, a very flexible structure, is less protected to allow for its extensive range of motion. It also supports the weight of the head via the bones of the neck (the cervical vertebrae), the ligaments that hold the bones together, and the muscles and tendons that support the structure. This combination increases its vulnerability to injury. The most predominant cause of pain is damage to the soft tissue of the neck—the muscles, tendons, and ligaments. Soft tissue damage can occur because of overuse or injuries such as whiplash and can manifest as sprains, strains, trigger points, and/or fascial tightening. It can also be secondary to abnormalities in the vertebrae, thus creating a pain-spasm-pain cycle. Abnormalities can be the result of birth defects, trauma from accidents (e.g., fractures, joint misalignments), degenerative and inflammatory diseases such as arthritis, or prolonged wear and tear resulting in cervical disk degeneration or protrusion (herniated disk). The thin, gelatinous material of the disk—the shock absorber between the vertebrae of our spine—degenerates as we grow older (typically age forty and up), creating less space between the bones and more friction. More friction creates pain that signals the soft tissue to initiate a splinting action (a spasm) to reduce further movement. This restriction only creates further pain, which perpetuates the pain-spasm-pain cycle. A herniated disk protrudes from between the vertebrae and causes pressure on the spinal cord or nerves, with resulting pain. Less frequently, neck pain can be caused by tumors or infection. Emotional stress is also an important contributing factor to perpetuating pain, especially since it slows the rate of improvement. Neck pain often causes or is a major contributor to headaches and shoulder, arm, and back pain. The longer a person has pain, the more effort is needed to correct it.

What Aggravates It?

As with low back pain, inactivity and dysfunctional biomechanics are primary aggravators of neck pain. With inactivity, the soft tissue becomes even more stiff and inflexible, decreasing the amount of circulation in the area which is necessary for a speedy recovery. Dysfunctional biomechanics further slows down recovery by either continuing the same habits and postures that created the pain in the first place or by further irritating an injury due to trauma or an asymmetry (defect) in the bone structure. Dysfunctional biomechanics would include postures or movements while standing, sitting, and sleeping. The head-forward, rounded-shoulder posture is a prime contributor to neck pain.

Fatigue and emotional stress both factor into the pain equation. Fatigue directly affects our sense of well-being. We are less prone to continuing our supportive postural habits and more inclined to slouched, contracted postures with the subconscious thought of conserving energy when, in reality, just the opposite occurs. Emotional stress, whatever its cause, creates further tightness in the soft tissue and can worsen existing neck tension.

Our environment may also play a role in neck pain. For instance, a cool draft on the neck can cause stiffness and discomfort. This is a frequent occurrence in the summer months, when people sleep with a fan blowing on them, or during seasonal changes, such as summer to autumn to winter. Other examples of environmental stressors are allergies, fumes or odors from smoke, paint, or some household cleaning products. These stressors may irritate our respiratory system and eyes, causing us to tense our muscles in the surrounding areas as a defensive mechanism.

Self-Help Measures

- If neck pain does not subside, or you experience tingling, numbness, or sharp, shooting pain referrals to other areas of your body, then schedule an appointment to see a medical professional, such as a chiropractor, orthopedic doctor, or physical rehabilitation specialist.
- Maintain supportive postural habits. Practice bringing your sternum up and contracting your lower abdominal muscles to bring your head and neck into better alignment while sitting or standing.
- If you wear eyeglasses, be sure your prescription is current or is adequate for your needs. If you spend large amounts of time at the computer, you may need special computer glasses.
- Speaking of computers, ideally the monitor should be 18 to 24 inches away, and the top line should be approximately at eye level.
- Strategic use of pillows to adequately support your neck while sleeping is necessary. There are pillows of all different types, shapes, and sizes, so experiment until you come up with the right combination. Sleeping on your stomach will increase neck pain because the neck stays in a rotated position.
- When reading, be sure to keep your light positioned so you can maintain an ideal posture without straining or rotating your neck.
- Keep the neck warm. In cooler weather this may mean wearing a turtleneck shirt even to bed!
- Use ice, heat, or both to alleviate pain and discomfort.
- Maintain gentle movements of the neck. Modify any stretching or other activities involving the neck to stay within your tolerance. There are also many people who specialize in movement therapies, such as Feldenkrais, Hanna Somatics, Continuum, and the Alexander method.

- Get some exercise even if it is just a walk around the block. The increased circulation and endorphin level will help reduce the pain and bring much-needed nutrients and oxygen to the area. Consult with a qualified professional for appropriate strengthening exercises when you are ready.
- Find ways to manage stress. Mental and physical flexibility are important.
- If your pain is related to conditions such as arthritis or fibromyalgia, there are support groups that may have information and tips on how to manage your pain.
- Massage therapy can greatly relieve soft tissue tension. If pain is due to disk degeneration or herniation, decreasing muscle tightness will help alleviate pain caused by the pain-spasm-pain cycle.

Stretching Recommendations

Practice the seven-minute neck and shoulder routines daily. Incorporate trunk and hip stretches a few times a week.

Thoracic Outlet Syndrome

What Is It?

Thoracic outlet syndrome (TOS) is a variety of symptoms caused by abnormal pressure on the neurovascular bundle between the neck and the lower end of the armpit—the thoracic outlet area. The neurovascular bundle refers to a group of nerves (the brachial plexus) and blood supply (subclavian artery and vein). This bundle supplies the fingers, hand, arm, shoulder girdle, and some regions of the head and neck with circulation. Nerve compression is more frequently involved than restriction of the blood supply. The most common symptoms are swelling or puffiness of the hand and fingers, dull achiness in the neck and shoulder region especially at night, fatigue in the arm, pain in the hand especially in the fourth and fifth fingers, tingling and numbness in the neck, shoulder, arm, and hand, and muscle weakness with difficulty gripping things and doing fine motor activities. These symptoms can also result from doing activities with the arm elevated, like combing or blow drying your hair or driving a car. The pressure is often created by tight muscles in the neck (the scalenes) and in the chest (the pectoralis minor). Its cause could also be from a narrowing of space between the collarbone, first rib, and soft tissue structures. This is usually due to poor bio-mechanics or carrying heavy loads. It is not common, but some people may be born with an extra rib above their first rib. This creates compression in the area because there is less room for all the structures.

What Aggravates It?

TOS often results from poor or strenuous postures, trauma, or static muscle tension in the shoulder area. Occupations that require repetitive movement and posture, such as cashiers, assembly line workers, plasterers, and electricians, are typically affected. It can also occur in people who stock shelves, catalogue books, or do needlework. Athletes who play volleyball, swimmers, tennis players, or baseball pitchers can all be affected. Musicians, particularly violinists, are also susceptible to this condition. Carrying heavy loads, children, briefcases, purses, and daypacks over one shoulder can aggravate TOS as well.

Self-Help Measures

It is important when you experience discomfort that suggests nerve involvement, such as numbness, tingling, puffiness, or other similar symptoms in the arms or legs, that you seek medical attention for an accurate diagnosis. There are other syndromes or medical problems that could have similar symptoms with different treatments. With that said, TOS responds well to manual therapy, such as massage or physical therapy and stretching exercises. It is also necessary for you to look at your activities of daily life to determine what postures or biomechanics need to be modified to alleviate the symptoms and make a more permanent change. Overall, TOS can be well-managed by taking the following measures:

- Sit erect with lumbar support. This keeps the shoulders back.
- Avoid sleeping on the affected side.
- Avoid folding or crossing your arms.
- Take breaks every fifteen to thirty minutes from repetitive work in which you bend slightly forward.
- Avoid lifting things above shoulder level.

Stretching Recommendations

Alternate daily between one or two of the seven-minute trunk, neck, shoulder, and arm routines.

Rotator Cuff Injury

What Is It?

This is a common injury of the shoulder. The rotator cuff refers to a group of four muscles and their tendons (tendons attach the muscles to bone) that hold the bones of the shoulder and the arm together. The muscles attach to the shoulder blade and the chest wall, and the tendons attach to the top of the arm (humerus). They provide the stability and support necessary for the shoulder joint's 360-degree rotation. Injuries occurring in the rotator cuff are due to direct trauma, such as a fall on or a blow to the shoulder, or trauma due to repetitive motion with a raised arm. Another cause of injury can be shoulder instability because of soft tissue looseness. Impingement is a term frequently heard in connection with a shoulder injury. It can occur after the initial trauma with resulting inflammation and swelling. This combination reduces the amount of space between the shoulder and the arm for the tendon to pass through, impinging on movement and, in most cases, causing pain. Other conditions associated with rotator cuff injury are tendinitis (inflammation of the tendon) and bursitis (inflammation of the bursa). The bursa is a fluid-filled sac that usually lies between the bone and the tendons, padding the soft tissue from friction and irritation. If the bursa becomes irritated (bursitis), it increases in size, creating less space and therefore more irritation, friction, and pain.

What Aggravates It?

Rotator cuff injury is caused by repetitive raised-arm movements, such as stocking shelves or writing on the blackboard; sports involving a swinging motion, such as baseball, tennis, swimming, ultimate frisbee, or riding the subway during rush hour and hanging on to the overhead strap; playing a musical instrument, such as the flute or violin; household activities, such as painting, scraping, vacuuming, window washing; and other similar activities.

Self-Help Measures

- Rest the area from strenuous activity but continue nonirritating movements.
- If the activity causes pain, then modify it.
- Avoid overhead movements for an extended period of time. For example, if you are painting or washing windows, use a ladder to keep movements below the shoulder.
- If you are vacuuming, keep the vacuum cleaner near your hip and walk as you vacuum rather than using an outstretched arm to move it.
- Do stretches while in the hot shower.
- When sleeping, use pillows to support the arm and shoulder so that it is not in an overstretched position.
- Try lying on a tennis ball to "work out" trigger points in the affected muscles.

- Try therapeutic massage or physical therapy.
- If you work at a computer, be sure the keyboard and mouse are in comfortable placement for your arm and shoulders.
- Modify your gym workouts to avoid lifting weights overhead if there is pain.
- Avoid propping your arm up on the door of the car or the console while driving so that your muscles are not in a shortened position. Also, shift your hand placement on the steering wheel from time to time.

Stretching Recommendations

Do daily seven-minute stretching routines of the neck and shoulders. Include the trunk, hip, and arm routines at least three times per week.

Tennis Elbow

What Is It?

Tennis elbow is known as lateral epicondylitis or, more simply, tendinitis. It is inflammation of the tendon attachment to the humerus that forms the bony protuberance on the outside part of the elbow (the epicondyle). The tendon is connected to the muscle that works the wrist and fingers. The pain involved usually begins at the outside of the elbow and can radiate down the arm and, in severe cases, to the hand. Most commonly, pain and sometimes weakness is brought on by grasping things like the steering wheel while driving or even picking up a glass. Sometimes an achy discomfort is present at night or after activities. Because we continually use our hands and arms, consistent care must be given to correct the injury.

A similar condition can occur on the inside or medial part of the elbow. It is called medial epicondylitis but is commonly known as golfer's elbow.

What Aggravates It?

Tendinitis is microtearing of the attachment site due to strong repetitive motion with the elbow extended and overloaded in sports like tennis, golf, or swimming. It can also result from any number of activities subject to repetitive stress, such as hammering, turning a screwdriver, computer work, excessive handshaking (politicians beware!), or window washing. It commonly occurs when the amount of activity has increased, or when poor conditioning or poor technique is involved.

Self-Help Measures

Reduce the pain and inflammation through rest, ice, compression, and elevation (more severe cases). This is a method called RICE, which we discuss later in the book.

To rest the area simply means modifying or avoiding the activities that aggravate the condition. It may mean modifying the grips on the golf clubs or tennis racquet and building up the grip on a screwdriver. Maintaining some movement of the affected area is necessary to promote circulation and tissue healing. Regular application of ice to the area will help control pain and discomfort and subsequently help reduce inflammation. Many people find a bag of frozen peas works well, since it readily conforms to the area and can be reused time and again. Leave it on for ten minutes and repeat three to four times throughout the day. For compression, use a forearm/elbow band to support the tendon attachment during activities. In more severe cases, wrap the area with an elastic bandage to aid in decreasing the swelling. Elevating the arm above the heart is suggested for severe swelling.

Soft tissue manipulation by a trained professional, such as a massage therapist or physical therapist, will help. With appropriate instruction from a physical or massage therapist, you can treat yourself with ice massage and deep transverse friction. Certain heat-producing liniments, available from an acupuncturist or herbalist, may bring relief by improving circulation to the area.

If these methods don't bring the relief you're looking for, several ultrasound treatments by a physical therapist often achieve a positive outcome.

As in all other conditions we have described, regular stretching can be very beneficial as a form of treatment and as prevention for recurring tendinitis.

Stretching Recommendations

Do a daily performance of the seven-minute shoulder and arm routines.

Carpal Tunnel Syndrome

What Is It?

Carpal tunnel syndrome (CTS) is the most common repetitive stress injury (RSI) or cumulative trauma disorder (CTD) seen by physicians, physical/occupational therapists, or massage therapists. It is also one of the most preventable conditions in this category. It presents as pain, burning, numbness, or tingling in the wrist or hand, which becomes worse after using the hands for activities requiring wrist action. This pain develops as a result of compression of the median nerve, which travels through a narrow "tunnel" where the wrist meets the palm. Nine tendons also pass through the carpal tunnel. When certain activities are performed that require sustained or repeated flexion, extension, or twisting of the wrist, friction occurs among the tendons in the carpal tunnel, which creates inflammation and swelling. This process of inflammation pushes on the median nerve, which affects much of the palm, thumb, index, middle, and ring fingers. Besides pain, tingling, and so on, carpal tunnel syndrome can lead to muscle weakness and a general impairment of hand function. For many individuals, the wrist/hand pain is worse at night, such that the numbness interrupts sleep.

Another factor that contributes to a narrowing of the tunnel besides inflammation is overly tight muscles of the forearm. The main movement of the fingers comes from the muscles of the forearm, up near the elbow. The attachment sites of these muscles are on the hand and fingers. With tight muscles, there is considerable pull exerted on their tendons/attachment sites. This pull can compress the bones of the wrist closer together, subsequently narrowing the carpal tunnel or increasing pressure on the wrist joint or finger joints. Couple this narrowing with friction among the tendons, and you have a painful condition which develops more quickly.

It is important to note that myofascial trigger points in the forearm or shoulder girdle can also bring on the same warning signs and mimic carpal tunnel syndrome. Unfortunately, we have seen individuals who had wrist/hand pain and went to their doctors, who immediately recommended surgery. After their surgical recovery, they still had pain and with further examination found that the cause of their pain was from a trigger point easily treated through massage or physical therapy. CTS responds well to noninvasive soft tissue manipulation. We believe surgery should only be the last resort after less invasive means have not produced results.

What Aggravates It?

Repetitive motion of the hands, wrist, or forearm certainly aggravates the symptoms of CTS. Gripping, grasping, or lifting with the thumb and index finger can strain the wrist. Sleeping positions that place the hand in extreme flexion (palm curled in) or extension (palm bent out) place considerable stress on the tendons of the carpal tunnel. Computer work, playing certain musical instruments, assembly line work (like twisting a screwdriver), and housework (scrubbing floors, sinks, and tubs) all contribute to strain on the tendons that pass through the tunnel. Previous bone fractures or dislocations in or around the wrist may produce a narrowing of the carpal tunnel and thus increase the risk for development of symptoms. Problems with fluid retention can also create swelling in the carpal tunnel and subsequently compress the median nerve.

Self-Help Measures

The most effective treatment program for CTS is prevention. Many of the repetitive activities that contribute to CTS overuse the flexor muscles of the forearm (inside of the forearm). These muscles become overly tight and compress the wrist joint and finger joints because of the pull on their long tendons, which cross the wrist. Counteracting the repetitive activity by stretching the forearm flexor muscles is of ultimate importance. This can be done any time or any place. It is also important to do the following:

- Keep the wrist in a neutral or straight position. To assist this at night, a wrist splint is helpful.
- Avoid repetitive movements or holding an object in the same way for extended periods of time.
- Reducing the speed with which you do a forceful, repetitive movement gives your wrist time to recover from the effort.
- Rest your hands periodically.
- Alternate easy and hard tasks, switch hands, or rotate work activities.
- Stretch, stretch, stretch.

The earlier you have a professional diagnosis and treatment, the more successful the outcome will be. Typical medical treatment begins with a splint, medication, or both. If symptoms continue, then surgery is recommended. This approach may calm the inflammation initially, but it's not treating the cause of the problem. In many patients choosing surgery, virtually all the symptoms return within three to five years as the ligaments within the carpal tunnel expand into the space created by the surgical division.

As mentioned earlier, repetitive activity causes muscles to tighten, shorten, harden, and grow inflexible. This muscle tightness can aggravate joints, cause nerve entrapment, and diminish blood flow and nutrient exchange to the affected tissues. Doing regular flexibility exercises can reverse this progression and eliminate, or at least better manage, symptoms of CTS. Soft-tissue manipulation or therapeutic massage by a skilled practitioner can loosen the hypercontracted muscles and allow stretching to be more effective. Vitamin supplementation with B_2, B_6, B_{12}, C, and folacin allows for improved tissue healing. Acupuncture has shown to be a very effective means for improving CTS.

All the mentioned self-help measures will be enhanced if the originally offending activity is modified or eliminated.

Stretching Recommendations

Doing the seven-minute arm/wrist and shoulder stretching routines daily is important for prevention and recovery. It's a good idea to include the seven-minute neck routine at least every other day.

Low Back Pain

What Is It?

Low back pain is among the five most common reasons for a physician visit in the United States. It is responsible for billions of dollars in health care costs and lost time at work each year. It is largely a preventable problem.

Mostly a musculoskeletal condition of overuse and improper body mechanics, low back pain may also be due to a less common disease process such as a tumor or dysfunction of an organ in the low back region.

The muscles of the back attach to the spine, the ribs, the hips, and all surrounding structures. As these muscles develop patterns of overuse or improper use, they become unusually tight on one side of the back or the other (or both sides). These patterns of tightness gradually increase over the years. With the back holding considerable chronic tension, it doesn't take much to "throw it out." In the case of an acute traumatic injury, these muscles may go into immediate spasm and cause extreme pain. As the muscles hold this tightness, they become less flexible and fatigue easily. They may entrap small nerves or nerve endings in the nearby area and send referred pain to another area of the body, such as into the hip and down the leg. This muscle tightness also creates greater pressure within the joints where they attach. For example, the muscles that attach to each vertebra of the spine will pull the vertebrae closer together as the muscles become tighter. This compression squeezes the intervertebral disks between the vertebrae and causes the disk to break down or wear unevenly. This can also place pressure on the spinal nerves, which can send referred pain down the leg as well. This spinal nerve compression with pain down the leg is known as sciatica. In our experience, it is more common to have low back pain and its resulting referred pain be related to trigger points or to tight muscles that entrap smaller nerves. Trigger points are areas in the muscle that are irritable from chronic tension or misuse and when touched or strained send a sensation of pain or discomfort to another part of the body.

Trigger points and nerve entrapments from tight muscles are easily remedied through massage, stretching, and some aerobic and strengthening activity. With persistent back pain, it is important to have a physician diagnose the extent of the problem. Oftentimes, however, medication, surgery, and/or bed rest is prescribed. If the condition is related to a ruptured or protruding disk then surgery may be necessary. Statistically, over 50 percent of all low back operations end up with similar pain problems. Surgery may relieve the pain by removing some or all of a disk, but it doesn't address what brought it on in the first place. Medication is useful for reducing pain and inflammation, but it does not treat the cause of the problem either. The original cause is due to tight muscles from improper body mechanics or overuse. Conventional medical wisdom says that bed rest is necessary for low back pain. Gordon Waddell, M.D., author of a recent systematic review on bed rest as treatment for back pain says, "Traditional management of back pain by rest is now discredited. . . . We no longer use bed rest to treat any other musculoskeletal condition." Authors of the British Guidelines on the Management of Acute Back Pain conclude, "For acute or recurrent low back pain with or without referred leg pain, bed rest for two to seven days is worse than placebo or ordinary activity." In general, bed rest is no longer recommended for any length of time unless lying down is the only position that does not elicit pain. Activity that is pain-free or minimally uncomfortable is preferable and may result in a faster recovery.

What Aggravates It?

Inactivity or dysfunctional biomechanics are the main factors that aggravate or instigate low back pain. That is, inactivity involving lack of movement (couch potato, sitting at a desk all day, etc.), lack of flexibility, lack of aerobic fitness, and lack of appropriate strength all contribute to vulnerable and weakened muscles of the back. Dysfunctional biomechanics is a term that includes improper posture, improper lifting, and improper movement patterns. Improper movement and posture can be due to the way the body has compensated for old injuries or can be related to stress and emotional strain.

Any time the trunk and head are tilted forward, even just leaning forward to hear someone speak or to write at a desk, the long muscles on either side of the spine are in a contracted state. This includes standing postures too. Bending forward with straight knees to rinse your mouth after brushing your teeth locks up the back muscles. Lying flat on your back without support under your knees can aggravate a sore back. Those "comfortable" positions we choose to stand in, with all the weight on one leg and the other foot twisted out in some other direction, favor muscles that are already too tight and can aggravate the back. Fatigue and overwork can certainly worsen back problems too.

Self-Help Measures

There are many things you can do to prevent or reduce low back pain. Overall, the best way to manage a low back problem is to have a balance between enough strength to do the activities of your daily living, adequate flexibility, and a good oxygen supply to your muscles through aerobic fitness. The other primary factors to consider are erect standing and sitting postures and good spinal alignment when lying on your side.

The following are just a few tips for preventing or taking charge of your back pain:

- Use lumbar support when sitting in a chair or automobile seat.
- Sit all the way to the back of the chair with your feet flat on the floor.

- Adjust the car seat back so that it is in the fullest upright position.
- Move the car seat closer to the steering wheel so your legs don't strain to reach the pedals.
- Place one foot up on the bumper when lifting something from the trunk of a car.
- Bend your knees when lifting.
- Avoid bending your back while lifting.
- If lifting something heavy, either get assistance or squat close to the object, hold it near your belly, and use your legs to bring your body to an upright position.
- Avoid twisting your body while lifting.
- Instead of leaning over a desk, use a clipboard to bring your work closer to you.
- Take frequent breaks from any position, every thirty minutes or so.
- Avoid leaning forward and reaching. When possible, position yourself so you are closer to your work.
- When sleeping on your back, place a pillow under your knees.
- When sleeping on your side, try to keep your spine straight. A "body pillow" may assist you from twisting and torquing your spine.
- Avoid sleeping on your stomach.
- Emergency relief position: in the event of severe back pain where there is no position of relative comfort, lie on your back on the floor and rest your legs (calves and feet) up on a chair or couch.

Ice vs. Heat

There are many opinions about icing and heating, and each of them seems to be strongly held. Some individuals have a constitution that cannot tolerate ice, and others cannot tolerate heat. If you are one that has a strong mental and physical reaction to ice or heat, let that be your guide as to which one you choose. In our experience, if there's an acute injury or spasm, ice is beneficial the first day or two in order to decrease the metabolic needs of the tissue and to interrupt the pain-spasm-pain cycle. After a couple of days, heat is relaxing and tends to bring more blood flow to the area.

Contrast therapy is perhaps the most effective form of hydrotherapy. This method uses both ice and heat and can be very beneficial after the initial injury is calmed down a bit or in the case of a backache. Try using moist heat on the area for three minutes and then one minute of ice, repeating this sequence for twenty minutes. This can be done in a bath by sitting in hot water three minutes, easing the affected area of the body out of the water for one minute of ice, then immersing another three minutes, and so on, for twenty minutes. Again, some people prefer one over the other, so if heat-ice-heat is irritating to you, try the opposite—ice-heat-ice.

Stretching Recommendations

Daily stretching with the seven-minute hip/low back routine is important for managing low back pain because of the pull these muscle groups have on the pelvis. Add the lower trunk stretching routine every other day.

Shinsplints

What Is It?

The term *shinsplints* has been commonly used to describe pain in the anterior or medial (front or inside) area of the lower leg. It can also be called medial tibial stress syndrome, periostalgia, or soleus syndrome. It is due to the pulling away of muscle fibers from the periosteum, the covering of the bone, and the bone itself. It is an overuse syndrome that usually develops over a gradual period of time; however, it can happen after just one incidence of strenuous exercise. It frequently occurs because of constant, rhythmic exercise, such as running or aerobics, and especially in inadequately conditioned athletes or new runners. In the early stages, the pain is usually relieved by rest. Pain in later stages often progresses in intensity and duration.

Another condition associated with shinsplints and lower leg pain is compartment syndrome. Each of the four compartments of the lower leg is comprised of muscles groups within a fascial "stocking"—anterior, lateral, superficial, and deep posterior. (Fascia is a tough, thin membrane of connective tissue covering the muscles.) The most commonly involved muscle groups are the anterior and deep posterior. Compartment syndrome refers to a condition in which pressure, due to inflammation, increases within the compartment because of restriction by the fascia and bone. This in turn puts pressure on the venous return of the blood (return of the blood back to the heart via the veins) and also on the nerves, thereby reducing circulation. The pain is often dull and achy with broad tenderness. Compartment syndrome, if left untreated, can have severe consequences.

What Aggravates It?

Most common in runners, shinsplints can occur in anyone taking on too much, too fast, without appropriate rest. (A good example would be a whirlwind sightseeing trip.) They can be aggravated by a change in running/walking style, terrain, or shoes. The sole of a shoe, either too flexible or too rigid, can be a culprit. Excessive pronation (wearing down the inside edge of the sole of your shoe) and/or abnormally loose subtalar joints (joints below the ankle) are also factors in this condition. Compartment syndrome can also be caused by blunt trauma, such as a kick to the shin in soccer. Early in its onset, the pain commonly begins later in the exercise and is relieved by rest. As shinsplints progress, the pain is usually worse in the beginning of exercise and then decreases during it, hence the term "running through the pain." However, it is often worse after exercise or the next day.

Self-Help Measures

Rest from the activity that causes the pain is the best treatment. This means a dramatic decrease in the intensity and duration of the activity. Return to exercise should be gradual, with plenty of rest allowed between the workouts for the necessary tissue repair. Icing the affected area for ten minutes after a workout will help decrease pain and inflammation. Mild stretching of the lower leg muscles is suggested to increase flexibility and help decrease reinjury. Massage is also very beneficial after cooldown from activity and pain has subsided. Proper footwear is important. Inspection of the soles can often give a clue as to wear patterns and indicate abnormal motion in one leg. A qualified shoe salesperson can help in this area. For acute compartment syndrome, on the other hand, medical attention is needed quickly.

Stretching Recommendations

Daily stretching with the seven-minute lower leg routine is very important. Add the hip/low back every other day to keep the entire lower extremity flexible.

Plantar Fasciitis

What Is It?

Plantar fasciitis, one of the most common causes of heel pain, is a result of microtears and inflammation of the plantar fascia, which is a broad band of connective tissue on the bottom of the foot. It attaches from the heel bone to the base of the toes, providing support to the arch of the foot, and plays an important role in the proper foot mechanics of walking or running. Normal tension is placed on the plantar fascia while standing or pushing off the ball of the foot and toes. Plantar fasciitis can occur as a result of an increase in activity level, change in terrain during exercise, excessive pronation of the foot, increase in weight (not as common), or loss of elasticity due to the aging process. The pain is most noticeable in the morning when taking your first step out of bed or after a long period of inactivity. The quality of pain is usually unyielding and sharp, and the first step can be excruciating. Walking on the affected foot often feels crab- or clawlike until the fascia warms up and can stretch comfortably.

What Aggravates It?

A number of different factors can contribute to plantar fasciitis, such as an increase in training, terrain, improper footwear, going barefoot, and tightness in the calf muscles and Achilles tendon.

Self-Help Measures

Treatment of plantar fasciitis is fairly simple, yet it may take six to twelve weeks or longer of consistent treatment for reduction of pain. Generally speaking, the longer the pain has been present and the more severe the symptoms, the longer it will take to resolve the condition.

Rest and/or change in activity are suggested. Decrease the distance or intensity of running or walking or, more effectively, switch to jogging in a pool or cycling to reduce the stress on the foot and calf muscles. Also, changing the terrain—for example, running or walking on grass instead of pavement—can make an enormous difference.

Proper shoes with good cushioning are very important in the reduction of plantar fasciitis discomfort. The pain tends to be more severe when one is barefoot or wears shoes with little or no padding in the sole. Orthotics (custom-made shoe inserts) may be needed to correct any structural differences in the foot or leg, although caution is needed since the rigid type of orthotic may be irritating to the plantar fascia.

Deep, specific massage in the calf muscles and the foot may be helpful in alleviating the pain. However, if deep massage does not reduce the pain it may be doing more harm than good. It may work best after a warm shower. Rolling a small ball (e.g., a golf ball or handball) under the foot works very well and is very easy to do during the day if you have a desk job or at night after work. It helps to continue to massage and loosen the foot. Stretching is an integral part of any massage routine.

- Icing the area for ten minutes will help reduce the pain and irritation.
- Stretching on a consistent, daily basis is critical to the success of resolving plantar fasciitis.

Stretching Recommendations

Daily stretching with the seven-minute lower leg routine is imperative. Add the hip/low back routine every other day to keep the entire extremity flexible.

Chapter 5

General Fitness Principles

Physical fitness is not only one of the most important keys to a healthy body, it is the basis of dynamic and creative intellectual activity. The relationship between the soundness of the body and the activities of the mind is subtle and complex. Much is not yet understood. But we do know what the Greeks knew: that intelligence and skill can only function at the peak of their capacity when the body is healthy and strong; that hardy spirits and tough minds usually inhabit sound gods.

—John F. Kennedy

As we have suggested thus far, fitness is not merely going to the gym or becoming an athlete. It involves balance of the whole being—our physical, mental, emotional, and spiritual selves. Managing stress, engaging in satisfying occupational and personal relationships, and adopting a positive outlook are important. So are gratifying leisure activities and being connected in some way to nature and our immediate environment. While all are vital to optimal mental and physical health, our focus in this chapter is on physical health.

Balanced physical fitness requires a blending of three basic components: (1) flexibility, (2) aerobic, and (3) strength training. To achieve good, balanced fitness, you really can't do one without the others. Now let's look at the reality of our modern lifestyle. Most of us seem to be engaged in sedentary work endeavors, and the rest of our lives are spent running around with numerous social and family commitments. The longer we sit at a desk or the more we lift the baby or some other repetitive activity, the shorter certain muscles become. The best fitness plan begins with increased flexibility. As the muscles become more flexible, joints develop a greater range of motion, and chances of injury from any fitness activities or daily lifestyle are dramatically reduced. As flexibility increases, so does vitality.

The emphasis in this book is on active-isolated stretching. We, the authors, both have been involved in some sort of physical fitness activity through much of our lives. As we have gained experience, the importance of a regular flexibility program has become more apparent to us. Various stretching methods have helped us maintain a certain level of flexibility. However, the active-isolated method is the only one that has allowed us to achieve a much improved flexibility without injury in the process.

Flexibility

Flexibility has been variously defined as mobilization, freedom to move, or, technically, the range of motion (ROM) available in a joint or group of joints. Stress, tension, repetitive motion activities, strength training, overuse or lack of use (couch potato) of certain muscles all shorten muscles and make them less flexible.

The flexibility exercises recommended in this book can function as warm-up for an average day as well as for strenuous activity and for a cooldown after a long day or physical workout. We recommend that an entire flexibility program from head to toe be practiced daily to bring balance and symmetry to the body. If your time is limited, spot stretching for the muscles most in need is appropriate. However, if all that you ever do is spot stretching, then you can easily create another set of imbalances over time. In the next chapter, we have outlined several seven-minute stretching routines that focus on various regions of the body.

Relaxation is probably the most important factor, other than stretching itself, in developing flexibility. Relaxation is the opposite of tension. Tension originates in contracted muscles, which result in inflexibility, insufficient oxygen supply (ischemia), and fatigue. In a flexibility training program it is important that you only stretch a relaxed muscle. Thus, your starting position and direction of movement is significant in order to avoid damage or microscopic tears in the muscle you are stretching. The active-isolated method described in this book addresses these concerns.

Benefits of a Flexibility Training Program—Why Stretch?

Stretching offers the following benefits:

1. It increases and maintains a joint's complete range of motion.
2. It relieves muscle soreness. Light exercise promotes a better supply of blood and oxygen to the muscles than complete rest and should be

pursued unless severity of injury to muscles or joints precludes further activity.

3. It improves capacity for activity. Stretched muscles require less energy for completion of movements. Contracted or tight muscles waste energy.
4. It promotes general body relaxation and reduces emotional stress.
5. It relieves muscle-joint stiffness associated with the aging process.
6. It increases musculotendinous elasticity. Muscle can be stretched 1.6 times its resting length before it tears.
7. It elongates the fascia, thereby improving posture and symmetry.
8. It helps prevent joint sprains, muscle strains or tears, and reinjury to previous joint and muscle trauma.
9. It reduces tightness, which may contribute to pain, spasm, or cramping.
10. It helps provide greater potentials of physical and athletic skills.
11. It provides an important adjunct toward recovery during the process of rehabilitation.
12. It offers a unique opportunity for spiritual growth by providing quiet intervals for thought, meditation, or self-evaluation. It's a great method to listen to your body.

Types of Stretching

Before we discuss the various types of stretching, it is important to note that flexibility can be developed at any age given the appropriate training. It's also interesting to note that, as a general rule, females are more flexible than males. The female is adapted for a greater range of flexibility, especially in the pelvic region, which accomodates pregnancy and childbearing. Specifically, because females have broader hips, they have a greater potential for range of motion.

Warm-up and Cooldown

Warm-up is important to help prevent muscle strain or tears from sudden over-lengthening of the musculotendinous unit. The primary purpose of a warm-up prior to physical activity is to raise the temperature deep within your body and to lengthen contracted muscle and fascial fibers. Warm-up also helps increase the speed of nerve impulses, which provides greater body movement potential. An older individual may require a longer warm-up.

Following vigorous exercise, slow your body's activity down gradually to allow your heart rate to return to the preexercise level. Although a cooldown may serve as an additional effort to improve flexibility (since the muscles are warm and well oxygenated), its main objective is to facilitate muscular relaxation, promote the removal of waste products, and reduce muscle soreness.

Active-Isolated Stretching

Active-isolated stretching may be used as an important part of warm-up, cooldown, or training for performance or rehabilitation. Specificity is important to achieve maximum circulation, relaxation, and tissue elongation. The muscles to be stretched should be identified and isolated by using precise, localized movements. The active-isolated stretch method involves contracting muscles opposite of those that are to be lengthened (agonist contracts, antagonist relaxes). The tissues to be lengthened are stretched for two seconds, and then the stretch is released. The area being stretched returns to the starting position, and this is repeated for the prescribed number of repetitions. Exhale during the stretching phase and inhale while returning to the starting position. Stretch the muscle only to the point of light irritation and then slowly release it to prevent a rebound contraction of the tissue you are stretching.

Ballistic Stretching

Ballistic stretching is usually associated with bobbing, bouncing, rebounding, and rhythmic motion. Often the terms isotonic, dynamic, kinetic, or fast stretching are used to refer to this kind of movement. The ballistic method tends to have potentially negative consequences, but in spite of this evidence there are still athletic teams that use this method as a "sport specific" benefit. Arguments against ballistic stretching include the following:

1. It tends to aggravate muscle and connective tissue because of the difficulty in judging the stretch tolerance of the tissues or failing to control the force of the body momentum.
2. It may create small muscle tears, which produce inflexible scar tissue.
3. It can often cause overtense muscles rather than produce relaxation.
4. It may initiate stretch reflex within the very muscles being stretched, causing rapid contraction of the muscles to be stretched and possible resulting spasms.

Ballistic stretching may be beneficial when training for specific athletic events that require a quick power start.

Static Stretching

In static stretching, you take the desired position and pull your body to the point where it can no longer go; then you gradually try to pull past that position for a few seconds—up to as long as one minute. The stretched part typically goes to a point of discomfort or pain and is gradually pushed beyond that point. Yoga is one example of static stretching. This method by itself is not safely effective for warm-up. Also, static stretching seems to facilitate the initiation of the stretch reflex by holding the stretch longer than three seconds, "moving past the pain," and causing a possible "rebound contraction." In other words, it's easy to overdo this method.

The Stretch Reflex

> *The stretch reflex is a regulatory mechanism of the nervous system that helps enable the body to maintain muscle tone and posture. It is activated as a defensive protection in an attempt to avoid overstretching and help prevent muscle/tendon injuries.*
>
> —Aaron Mattes

When there is not adequate flexibility for a required movement, the stretch reflex contraction exerts force against the desired movement. It is believed that the stretch reflex is activated in three to five seconds. Thus, with the active-isolated method of stretching, it is important to only hold the stretch two seconds so that the stretch reflex doesn't initiate a rebound contraction, creating a tug-of-war in the muscle being stretched.

Proponents of static stretching maintain that if the stretch is held long enough (twenty-five to thirty seconds) the stretch reflex will be inactivated, and then the muscle will be able to lengthen. Our concern is what may happen between three and thirty seconds. With the little tug-of-war going on, there is a much larger risk of microscopic tears or greater injury in the muscle being stretched.

Passive Stretching

Passive stretching is useful if you have a paralysis or soft-tissue injury. The motion or stretch is performed by an outside factor. This may either be a partner or special traction equipment. If joint range of motion (ROM) is not maintained following problems such as a stroke or spinal cord injury, the musculotendinous unit will shorten and joint motion will be affected. Passive stretching should be a slow, steady movement that gently lengthens the soft tissues. Careful movement of the tissues will help prevent pain. Ballistic motion or bouncing is not advised for extremely weak or paralyzed muscles, as rapid movement may activate the stretch reflex. Rapid movement will cause pain and increase the possibility of muscle or tendon rupture.

Proprioceptive Neuromuscular Facilitation (PNF)

One type of PNF is a partner-assisted stretching that can bring about relatively quick, short-term gains in flexibility. Proper completion of this PNF stretch involves a sequence beginning with a resisted isometric contraction that ends with an assisted stretch. Proprioceptive neuromuscular facilitation is an umbrella term for several types of contract-relax stretches. It is beneficial for rehabilitation settings and pre- and postathletic events for quick flexibility gains. The following is a typical contract-relax sequence:

1. Actively move the muscle to be stretched (target muscle) into a fully lengthened position without pain (end point).
2. Isometrically contract the target muscle against the resistance of a partner, using 20–30 percent of your strength, and hold this contraction about eight seconds.
3. Slowly relax this resisted contraction and bring the target muscle into a further stretch. Your partner will assist stretching the target muscle to a new end point if necessary.
4. Repeat the contract-relax-stretch cycle three to four times.

Aerobic Conditioning

You can begin aerobic conditioning almost simultaneously or soon after your muscles become more flexible. During aerobic activity, the muscles are getting their energy from oxygen. Therefore, aerobic activities are an excellent way to pump oxygen into tight and tired tissues. The other reason to be aerobically fit is to improve your cardiovascular fitness.

What Activities Are Aerobic?

To be aerobic, an activity needs to be rhythmic and continuous over at least twenty minutes. It also needs to involve a large percentage of the body's muscle mass. This includes walking, jogging, swimming, cycling, and rowing. Golf and football are not aerobic because of their stop-start nature. Singles tennis can be aerobic if it's a good game, while doubles is not. Walking the dog may not be aerobic if your dog pauses frequently for fire hydrants.

Of course, if you are just beginning an aerobic program and have a history of any serious health condition, check with your health care provider. Otherwise, here's a way to begin:

- If you're walking, purchase a supportive pair of walking or running shoes and use them only for your aerobic exercise. This helps protect your ankle, knee, and hip joints.
- Avoid walking during the hottest or coldest parts of the day.
- During the first month or so, choose to walk on relatively flat areas. Hills require more energy from your heart and joints.

- Walk slowly as you warm up for five minutes.
- Increase your speed for the next 20 minutes. One rule of thumb is if you are able to sing while walking, you need to walk faster, and if you find it difficult to carry on a conversation, you'd better slow down.
- Walk slowly for the next five minutes.
- It's a good idea to stretch before and especially after aerobic activity.
- Do this activity three to five times weekly, and increase your distance and speed over a few months.

If you have been ill or are considerably out of shape, begin walking only ten minutes. Increase by five minutes every week so you can follow the suggestions listed above. Monitoring your increase in exercise is important to avoid injury.

One can still gain some aerobic benefit if 25 or 30 minutes are not available in one chunk. If you can walk for ten minutes three or four times daily, you can reap some of the benefits that you would gain from a sustained thirty-minute walk. However, this method is more beneficial for burning fat than significantly increasing aerobic capacity.

Target Heart Rate

You can monitor how hard you are working by finding your perceived exertion or target heart rate. Perceived exertion simply means that if it feels like you are working hard, sweating and/or walking fast enough, then you are in the correct aerobic range. The other method is by monitoring your target heart rate. For a healthy individual, optimal aerobic benefit can be achieved by exercising between 60 percent and 85 percent of your capacity. Your target heart rate is measured by counting your pulse while exercising. It should be in the 60–85 percent range for at least twenty minutes. Use the five minutes before to warm up to this rate and the five minutes after to cool down to your resting heart rate.

The most accurate method of checking your pulse (heart rate) is to count it for a full minute, which shows how fast your heart is beating each minute. The most accurate way to check your resting heart rate (RHR) is before you get out of bed in the morning. During exercise, it's a good idea to stop and count your pulse for only ten seconds. If you count longer, your heart rate will probably drop out of your true exercise range. The target heart rate (THR) example shows how to determine the number of beats you should count in ten seconds. You can calculate your target heart rate (THR) using the following formulas:

THR = 220 − your age − your RHR × 60% (or .6) + your RHR
    (your heart rate should be above this number during exercise)

THR = 220 – your age – your RHR × 85% (or .85) + your RHR (your
heart rate should be below this number during exercise)

Example

A 25-year-old man has a resting heart rate of 65. To determine the lower end
of his target heart rate, subtract his age (25) from 220 (220 – 25 = 195); then
subtract his RHR of 65 (195 – 65 = 130). Now multiply this number by 60 percent (130 × .6 = 78), and then add the RHR (78 + 65 = 143). To calculate the
upper end of his target heart rate, do the same procedure, only multiply by 85
percent (.85). In this case, he will achieve maximum aerobic benefit while exercising with his heart rate between 143 and 175.

Lower End of Target Heart Rate	Upper End of Target Heart Rate
220	220
− 25 (age)	− 25 (age)
195	195
− 65 (RHR)	− 65 (RHR)
130	130
× .60	× .85
78	110
+ 65 (RHR)	+ 65 (RHR)
143	175

For a ten-second count, the heart rate should be between 24 and 29 (143 and
175 divided by 6).

Injury Prevention

Twenty to forty-five minutes of aerobic activity in your recommended target
heart rate range three to five times weekly is desirable. Keep in mind that most
exercise injuries occur with an increase of intensity or duration. So, if you are
accustomed to walking a mile in 20 minutes and are having a good day and
choose to walk that mile in fifteen minutes, be aware that you are at higher
risk for injury. You are at even higher risk if you choose to walk faster and
twice as long, say 40 minutes. Gradual build-up is the best way to proceed.
Another caution: if you are at a particular level of exercise and then become
sick with some flu bug for a week, pay attention. When you resume your aerobic activity, start at a much lower intensity and duration and allow your stamina to rebuild over a few weeks. Attention to these little details will keep you
off the injured list!

RICE

Rest the injured area.
I ce the injured area.
Compress the injury to prevent excessive swelling (e.g., wrap it with an elastic bandage).
Elevate the injured body part.

Should you become injured, the suggested protocol is RICE (see box) for the first 24 to 48 hours while signs of heat, pain, swelling, or redness are present. After signs and symptoms of inflammation have subsided, you may find relief by using a contrast of ice-heat-ice. A general rule of thumb is not to leave either the ice or heat on for any longer than ten minutes. Opinions vary about the order of ice and heat and how long to use each one. For example, some people prefer heat-ice-heat (3 minutes-1 minute-3 minutes), while others like ice-heat-ice (10 minutes-10 minutes-10 minutes). Your goal is to interrupt the pain cycle. Another benefit is that this alternation improves circulation to the area. Ice constricts the blood vessels while heat dilates them, which produces a type of pumping action. In effect, you are allowing the ice and heat to massage the area.

Strength Conditioning

Building strength should come after your flexibility starts to improve and your aerobic capacity expands. Lifting weights and using weight machines are excellent methods to create better muscle tone. So it is important when undertaking a strength-building program to also incorporate a stretching and aerobic fitness plan, to maintain the body at its optimum level of performance.

With any soft-tissue injury, there is usually considerable tightness in all the surrounding muscles to protect the area from further damage. If strength training is introduced before the tissues have reached appropriate elasticity, further limitations could likely result. An effective sequence during recovery from most soft-tissue injuries includes the elimination of spasms and hypercontraction of the tissues by some form of soft tissue therapy, the restoration of flexibility through stretching, and the gentle rebuilding of strength and endurance through aerobic conditioning. In a rehabilitation situation, the strength training and aerobic conditioning are nearly simultaneous. The therapy and stretching also go hand in hand.

Unless your goal is to enter bodybuilding competition, we advocate that strength conditioning involve light weights and more repetitions. Try to consider which muscles you use routinely and make sure the opposite muscles become strengthened as well. For example, if your daily activities involve lifting or working with your arms in front of you, your chest muscles are already getting quite a workout. Thus, it is important to strengthen the opposite muscles, the ones between your shoulder blades, to bring more balance to the area.

As with aerobic fitness, most strength conditioning injuries occur with increased intensity and duration. So gradually build any weight increases and the length of your workout. Most fitness facilities have qualified trainers to assist in the process.

The Effects of Aging on Muscle

With the normal aging process, there is barely any decrease in normal muscle function. This includes muscular strength, endurance, agility, and flexibility. This is in contrast to the "typical" aging process. What is typical in our society is not normal. Typically we see a decline in function due to inactivity and poor health practices. When complicated by disease or injury, these functions decline rapidly.

Physiologically, one of the most conspicuous degenerative changes associated with aging (as a result of inactivity) is the progressive atrophy, or wasting away, of muscle mass. This is due to both the reduction in size and number of muscle fibers. As muscle fibers atrophy, fatty and fibrous (collagen) tissue replacement occurs. Collectively, these changes appear to be partly responsible for the typical age-related loss of flexibility. This can be reversed successfully to a noticeable degree.

How many times have you heard someone say, "If I'd known I was going to live this long, I would have taken better care of myself"? It's never too late to begin a fitness program. If you are quite deconditioned, then the process of restoring flexibility and fitness needs to begin more slowly. You will notice your gains over the months instead of weeks. But since the introduction of cardiac rehabilitation exercise programs in the early 1980s, it has been demonstrated repeatedly that people with heart disease in their sixties and seventies can become more fit and feel more healthy than they have since their teens or twenties. It takes a commitment and deliberate plan of regular activity. Becoming more flexible is a great place to begin. Remember, if you don't use it, you lose it.

Chapter 6

How to Become
More Flexible the
Active-Isolated Way

Nothing happens until something moves.

—Albert Einstein

We made comparisons between various stretching methods in the last chapter. What makes the active-isolated method unique is the principle of reciprocal innervation. Other stretching methods attempt to stretch groups of muscles and muscles that are in an elongated contraction. With active-isolated stretching, you identify and isolate the muscle you want to stretch. Then you contract its opposite and actively move in a direction that provides a stretch. When one muscle of an opposing pair is contracted, the other one relaxes. Thus, a relaxed muscle is being stretched. This provides a better and safer stretch with much less opportunity for injury.

Reciprocal Innervation/Inhibition

Muscles usually operate in pairs so that when one set of muscles, the agonist, is contracting, the opposing antagonist set of muscles is relaxing. This grouping of coordinated and opposing agonist and antagonist muscles is called reciprocal innervation. Therefore, when one muscle is innervated or receives an impulse to contract, its opposite is inhibited and therefore relaxed. Active-isolated stretching operates on the same principle of reciprocal innervation/inhibition. In order to stretch a relaxed muscle, its action must be inhibited by contracting or innervating the opposing muscle. For example, when lifting a glass of water to your mouth, you must bend your elbow, thereby shortening, contracting, and innervating your biceps muscles. In order for this to happen, the impulses to the opposite muscles, the triceps, must be inhibited so they will stretch and lengthen to accommodate the shortening contraction of the biceps muscles.

When to Stretch

You can stretch anytime! For general balance with the major muscles of the body, we recommend that you use the entire head-to-toe stretching routine daily. If your schedule won't allow for the full routine, which may take thirty or forty minutes, choose the stretches that apply to the type of activities you'll be doing on a particular day. For your convenience, we have outlined several seven-minute stretching segments in the following section, which focus on various regions of the body. We have also outlined stretching routines suited for various activities. Stretching in the morning is a splendid idea, for it will prepare you for what you might face during the day. Think of stretching as your warm-up for the day.

Stretching in the middle of a specific activity to counteract potential overuse problems can be important. For example, while doing computer work, it's a good idea to take a few minutes' break at least every thirty minutes to briefly stretch the neck, shoulders, and arms. After doing a particularly heavy or repetitive activity, stretching can serve to act as your "reset button" and help prevent stiffness or soreness the next day. If you are on the job and time is critical, even stretching as little as one minute per hour will make a significant difference to your body in the long run.

No special equipment is needed. Certain leg stretches can be done more effectively with the assistance of an eight-foot length of rope, or towels, belts, or neckties tied together.

The positive changes should begin to appear within a couple of weeks. After several months, you most likely will notice that certain activities are easier and some body parts that were painful are no longer as bothersome.

Seven-Minute Stretching Routines

Neck Routine (sitting, standing, or lying down)
Flexion
Lateral Flexion
Rotation
Extension

Shoulders/Arms Routine
Horizontal Abduction Stretch
Backward Extension

Internal (Medial) Rotation
External (Lateral) Rotation
Straight Arm Lift/Pull Down
Sideward Arm Lift
Triceps Stretch
Biceps Stretch

Wrists/Hands Routine
Supination
Pronation
Wrist Flexors
Finger Flexors
Wrist Extensors
Finger Extensors

Lower Trunk Routine
Forward Trunk Bend
Twisting Trunk Bend
Pelvic Tilt
Hip Hiker
Knee to Opposite Shoulder
Thoracic Lift
Iliopsoas
Side Bends

Hip/Low Back Routine
Straight Leg Hamstrings
Quadriceps
Tensor Fascia Latae
Figure Four
Adductors

Lower Leg Routine
Gastrocnemius
Soleus
Tibialis Anterior
Inversion
Eversion
Metatarsal stretch

While it is preferable that you do a full-body stretching routine on a regular basis, sometimes there just isn't enough time in the day. Here are some suggestions for you on how to organize a specific seven-minute routine according to your daily activities. We have developed some basic routines for various regions of the body. For example, if your daily routine involves sitting at a desk or working on a computer, it would be most beneficial to do the shoulder and neck and hands routine several times a week and to add the low back routine when you have more time.

Take a typical day and examine your movements that occur most frequently. Look at the movements during your daily activities around the house, during work or recreation, sports, and hobbies. Determine which muscles are affected the most by your activities and focus on them, but not to the exclusion of other areas because, as we all know, no one part of the body works independently of the others. When there is a particular action in one part of the body, there is a ripple effect throughout the rest of the body.

Here are some suggestions to help you identify and prioritize your seven-minute stretching routines. The activities we have listed are examples to give you ideas for customizing your own personal program.

Daily Activities

Driving: neck, shoulders/arms, and hips/low back
Vacuuming: shoulders/arms and hips/low back
Doing yard work: shoulders/arms, lower trunk, and hips/low back
Lifting: shoulders/arms, lower trunk, and hips/low back
Using phone: neck and shoulders/arms

Sports/Recreation

Swimming: neck, shoulders/arms, lower trunk, and hips/low back
Cycling: neck, shoulders/arms, hips/low back, and lower legs
Running/walking/jogging: lower trunk, wrists/hands, hips/low back, and lower legs
Playing tennis: shoulders/arms, wrists/hands, hips/low back, and lower legs
Playing golf: shoulders/arms, lower trunk, and hips/low back

Occupations

Desk/computer worker: neck, shoulders/arms, wrists/hands, and hips/low back
Cashier: shoulders/arms, wrists/hands, lower trunk, and hips/low back
Mechanic: neck, shoulders/arms, wrists/hands, lower trunk, and hips/low back
Nurse: shoulders/arms, wrists/hands, and hips/low back
Teacher: neck, shoulders/arms, wrists/hands, and hips/low back
Musician: neck, shoulders/arms, wrists/hands, and lower trunk

Hobbies

Needlework/sewing: neck, shoulders/arms, wrists/hands, and hips/low back
Model-building: neck, shoulders/arms, wrists/hands, and hips/low back
Woodworking: shoulders/arms, wrists/hands, and hips/low back
Watching television: neck, lower trunk, and hips/low back

Active-Isolated Stretching: Important Considerations

1. Breathe freely and deeply. Exhale while performing the stretch and inhale while returning to the starting position.

2. Most of these stretches isolate a few muscles. Stretch only those muscles. Don't get your entire body in the act to get that extra inch or two.

3. Be mindful of proper body alignment. Stand with your feet pointing straight ahead, even with each other, and hip-width apart. Stand erect, as if a sky hook were pulling you slightly upward. Another description would be to stand with your sternum (breastbone) up and your lower abdomen and buttocks tucked in.

4. Hold each stretch for only two seconds.

5. If you are just beginning a flexibility program, start with only four to six repetitions of each exercise. Increase by two repetitions every week or two for a maximum of ten repetitions.

6. If something is painful, stop or reposition yourself. Only stretch to the point of light irritation: no pain is your gain. It may be that other muscles need to loosen before you can comfortably perform a particular stretch. So put the painful stretches on hold for several weeks; then reintroduce them gently and with only a few repetitions.

Active-Isolated Stretches

Neck Stretches: Sitting or Standing

These exercises can be performed while you are standing, sitting, or lying down. The standing and lying positions are illustrated. The lying stretches are more advanced and should be performed with caution or not at all for people with any disk problem (e.g., fusion, stenosis, arthritis). We have included these stretches because of their strengthening potential.

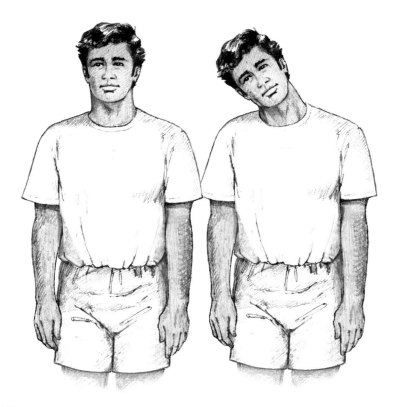

Lateral Flexion
Starting position: Stand or sit in a correct posture. Look straight ahead. Inhale. **Action:** While exhaling, lower your ear toward your shoulder, keeping a straight line. Stretch to light irritation and hold for two seconds. Inhale while you return to the starting position. Repeat four to ten times, depending on your fitness level. Repeat on the other side.

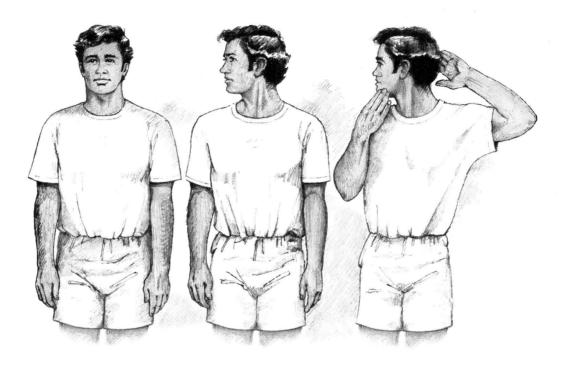

Rotation

Starting position: Stand or sit in a correct posture. Look straight ahead. Inhale. **Action:** While exhaling, rotate your chin over one shoulder and look behind. Be sure your shoulders face forward and only your head rotates. Stretch to light irritation and hold for two seconds. Inhale while you return to the starting position. Repeat four to ten times, depending on your fitness level. Repeat on the other side.

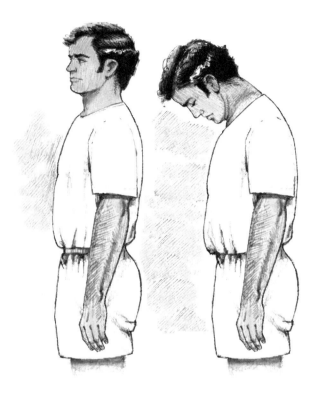

Forward Flexion
Starting position: Stand or sit in a correct posture. Look straight ahead. Inhale. **Action:** While exhaling, tuck your chin and roll your head down. Stretch to light irritation and hold for two seconds. Inhale while you return to the starting position. Repeat four to ten times, depending on your fitness level.

Neck Stretches: Lying

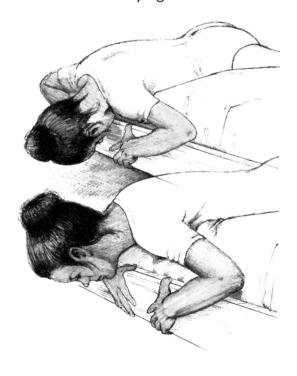

Extension
Starting position: Lie on your stomach with your arms and head hanging off the edge of the bed. Inhale. **Action:** While exhaling, lift your head up to neutral, parallel to the floor. Hold for two seconds. Inhale while you return to the starting position. Repeat four to ten times, depending on your fitness level.

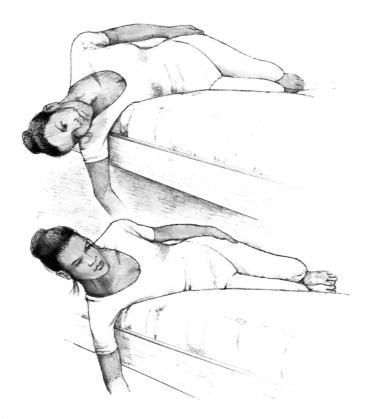

Lateral Flexion

Starting position: Lie on your side with your arm hanging over the edge of the bed and let your head hang freely toward the floor. Inhale. **Action:** While exhaling, bring your ear up toward your shoulder without twisting your head or moving your shoulder. Stretch to light irritation and hold for two seconds. Inhale while you return to the starting position. Repeat four to ten times, depending on your fitness level. Remain on this side and do the next stretch, the neck rotation.

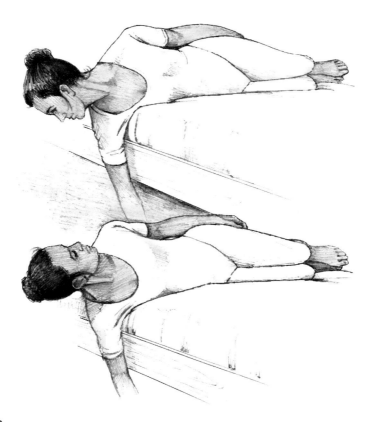

Rotation

Starting position: Lie on your side with your arm hanging over the edge of the bed keeping your head in straight alignment with your spine throughout this exercise. Rotate your head down so you look at the floor. Inhale.

Action: While exhaling, rotate your head and look up at the ceiling. Be sure your shoulders stay in a straight line and only your head is rotating. Stretch to light irritation and hold for two seconds. Inhale while you return to the starting position. Repeat four to ten times, depending on your fitness level. Repeat both the lateral flexion and the rotation on the other side.

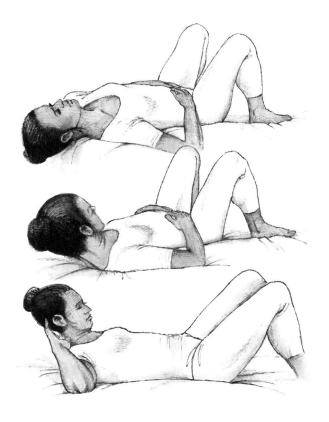

Forward Flexion

Starting position: Lie on your back. Inhale. **Action:** While exhaling, tuck your chin and roll your head toward your chest. Stretch to light irritation and hold for two seconds. Gently assist with your hands if further stretch is needed. Inhale while you return to the starting position. Repeat four to ten times, depending on your fitness level.

Shoulder, Arm, and Wrist Stretches

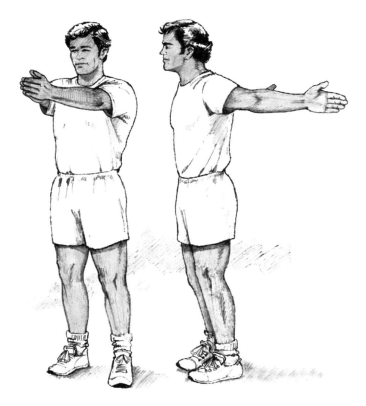

Horizontal Abduction

Starting position: Stand erect with your feet shoulder-width apart. Lift your arms to shoulder height, keeping them straight and parallel to the floor with palms together. Inhale. **Action:** Exhale while drawing shoulder blades close together, thus pulling your arms back as far as possible. Stretch to light irritation. Hold for two seconds and inhale while you return to the starting position. Repeat four to ten times, depending on your fitness level.

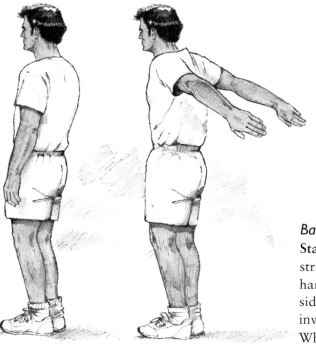

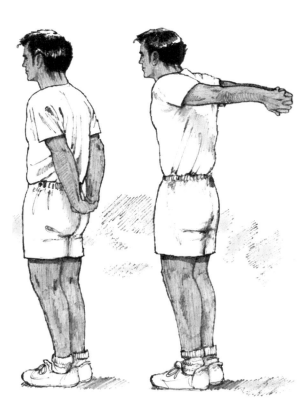

Backward Extension
Starting position: Stand straight with your arms hanging freely at your sides, palms facing inward. Inhale. **Action:** While exhaling, raise your straight arms and hands behind you while keeping your shoulders down and trunk straight. Stretch to light irritation. Hold for two seconds and inhale while you return to the starting position. Repeat four to ten times, depending on your fitness level. For a more advanced stretch, let your arms hang straight down with your hands clasped behind you and resting against your buttocks. Stretch as described above. Another variation is to do this with slightly bent elbows to access different muscle fibers.

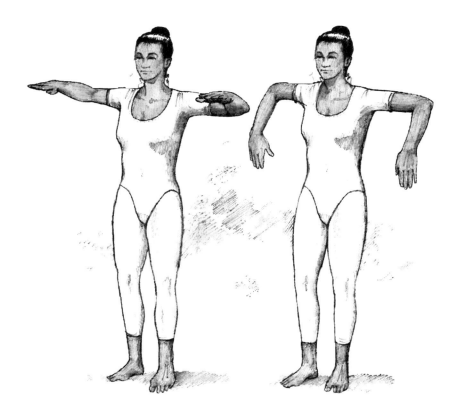

Internal Rotation

Starting position: Extend your arms out to the side and up to shoulder height. Bend your forearms to a 90-degree angle, palms facing down (have the image of a pole running though your shirt sleeves against your back at shoulder level). Inhale. **Action:** Exhale while lowering your forearms down and back as far as you can, keeping your elbows at shoulder height. Stretch to light irritation and hold for two seconds. Inhale while you return to the starting position. Repeat four to ten times, depending on your fitness level.

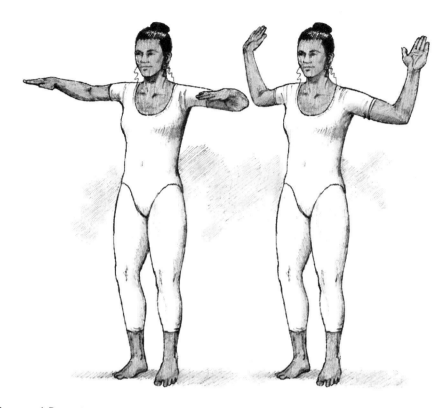

External Rotation

Starting position: Extend your upper arms out to the side and parallel to the floor and bend your forearms to a 90-degree angle, palms facing down (have the image of a pole running though your shirt sleeves against your back at shoulder level). Inhale. **Action:** Exhale while raising your forearms up and back as far as you can, keeping your elbows at shoulder height. Stretch to light irritation and hold for two seconds. Inhale while you return to the starting position. Repeat four to ten times, depending on your fitness level.

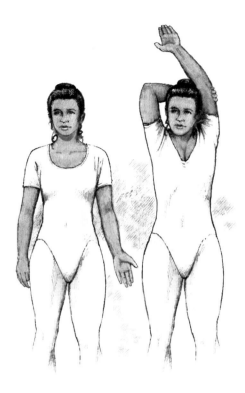

Sideward Arm Lift

Starting position: Stand straight with your feet shoulder-width apart and your arms hanging freely at your sides. Inhale. **Action:** While exhaling, turn the palm of your left hand forward, keeping your arm straight. Reach your arm out to the side and up as far as possible, bringing it behind your head. Assist the stretch by clasping your elbow with the opposite hand. Stretch to light irritation and hold for two seconds. Inhale while you return to the starting position. Repeat four to ten times, depending on your fitness level. Repeat for your other arm.

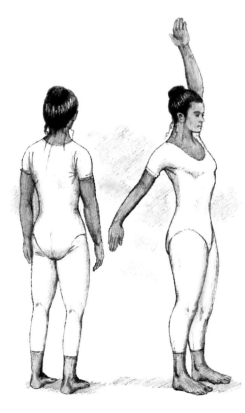

Straight Arm Lift Up/Pull Down

Starting position: Stand straight with your feet shoulder-width apart and your arms hanging straight at your sides, palms facing your body. Inhale. **Action:** While exhaling, and with elbows straight, reach one arm forward and up as far as possible while reaching the other arm down and back as far as possible. Do not twist your torso or arch your back. Stretch to light irritation and hold for two seconds. Inhale while your arms pass each other. Repeat four to ten times, depending on your fitness level.

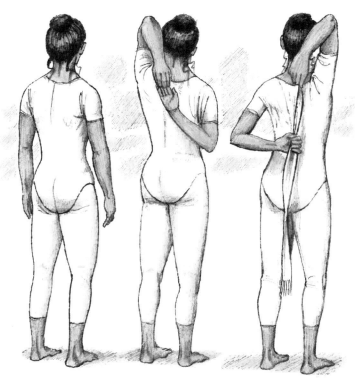

Posterior Hand Clasp

Starting position: Stand straight with your feet shoulder-width apart and your arms hanging freely at your sides. Inhale. **Action:** While exhaling, bring your left arm up so that your elbow points toward the ceiling and your hand dangles between your shoulder blades. At the same time, bring your right hand down behind your back and then up between your shoulder blades toward the left hand. If possible, clasp hands and stretch to light irritation. A rope or towel may be used to assist this movement. Hold on to the towel with both hands and slowly inch them toward each other. Hold for two seconds and inhale while you return to the starting position. Repeat four to ten times, depending on your fitness level. Repeat for your other arm.

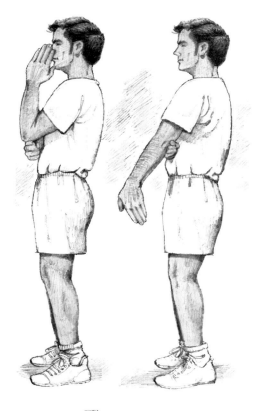

Biceps

Starting position: Stand straight with your right forearm bent, fingers pointing up and the palm facing your body's midline. Rest your left fist on your right hip, and then rest the right elbow on that fist. Inhale. **Action:** While exhaling, lower your right forearm to full extension, pulling the wrist and hand back even farther. Stretch to light irritation and hold for two seconds. Inhale while you return to the starting position. Repeat four to ten times, depending on your fitness level. Repeat for your other arm.

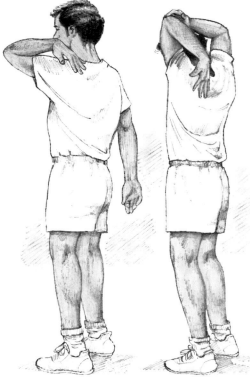

Triceps

Starting position: Bring your elbow up until the upper arm is shoulder height with your hand dangling over your shoulder. Inhale. **Action:** While exhaling, raise your elbow up toward the ceiling as your hand moves downward on the shoulder blade. Assist stretch with opposite hand. Stretch to light irritation and hold for two seconds. Inhale while you return to the starting position. Repeat four to ten times, depending on your fitness level. Repeat for your other arm.

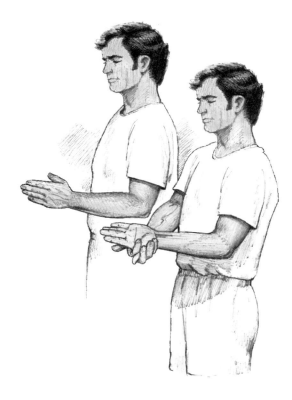

Forearm Supination/Pronation

Starting position: With your elbow at a 90-degree angle, tuck it against your side with your palm facing midline. Inhale.

Stretch A Supination stretches the pronator muscles of the forearm, which are used in activities such as throwing and racquet sports. **Action:** While exhaling, rotate the palm up and away from midline. Assist the stretch by placing your opposite hand on the back of the stretching hand. Stretch to light irritation and hold for two seconds. Inhale while you return to the starting position. Repeat four to ten times, depending on your fitness level. Repeat for your other arm.

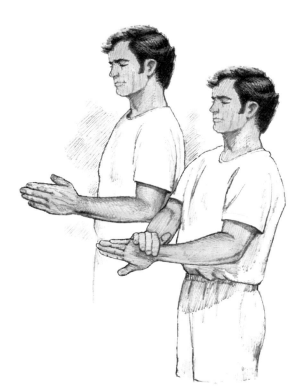

Stretch B Pronation stretches the supinator and biceps muscles of the arm, which are used in activities such as throwing and racquet sports. **Action:** Rotate the palm toward midline and down (thumb down). Assist the stretch by placing your opposite hand on the back of the stretching hand. Stretch to light irritation and hold for two seconds. Inhale while you return to the starting position. Repeat four to ten times, depending on your fitness level. Repeat for your other arm.

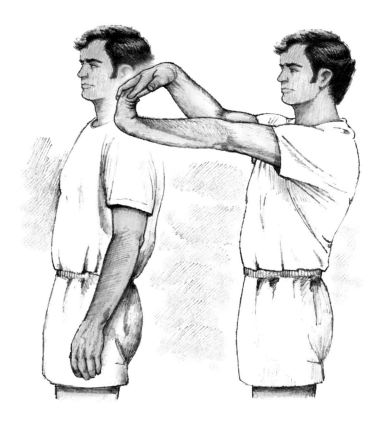

Wrist Flexor

Starting position: Standing straight, let your arms hang freely at your sides. Inhale.

Stretch A This stretches the flexors of the forearm and wrist, which are often involved in carpal tunnel syndrome. **Action:** While exhaling, raise your straight arm forward and up to shoulder level, palm down. Move the hand up into a "stop" position (palm out). Assist the stretch by using your opposite hand. Stretch to light irritation and hold for two seconds. Inhale while you return to the starting position. Repeat four to ten times, depending on your fitness level. Repeat for your other arm.

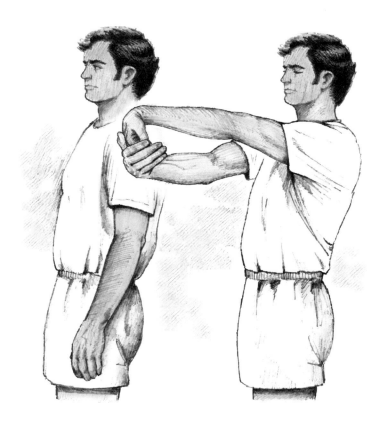

***Stretch B* Action:** While exhaling, raise your straight arm forward and up to shoulder level, palm up. Move the fingertips down so the palm faces forward. Assist the stretch by using your opposite hand. Stretch to light irritation and hold for two seconds. Inhale while you return to the starting position. Repeat four to ten times, depending on your fitness level. Repeat for your other arm.

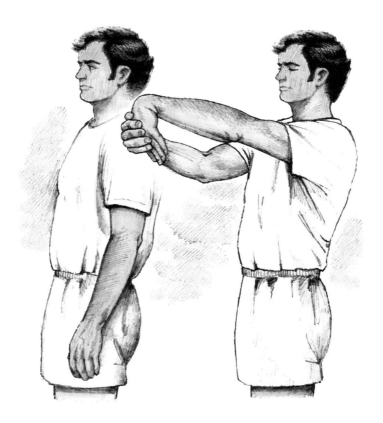

Wrist Extensor

Starting position: Stand erect with your arms hanging freely at your sides. Inhale. **Action:** While exhaling, raise your straight arm forward and up to shoulder level, palm down. Move your fingertips down so the palm faces back. Assist this stretch by using your opposite hand. Stretch to light irritation and hold for two seconds. Inhale while you return to the starting position. Repeat four to ten times, depending on your fitness level. Repeat for your other arm.

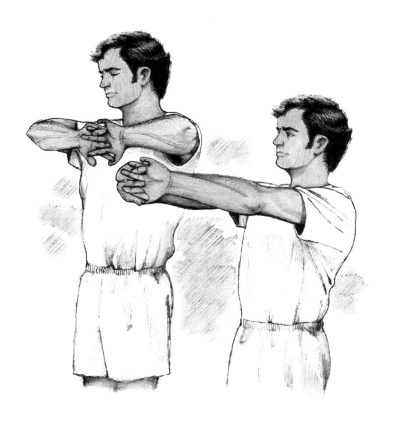

Finger Flexor

Starting position: With your hands at chest level, interlace the fingers so your palms are facing forward and the back of your hands touch your chest. Inhale. **Action:** While exhaling, straighten your arms so that the palms push forward and the fingers flatten out. Stretch to light irritation and hold for two seconds. Inhale while you return to the starting position. Repeat four to ten times, depending on your fitness level.

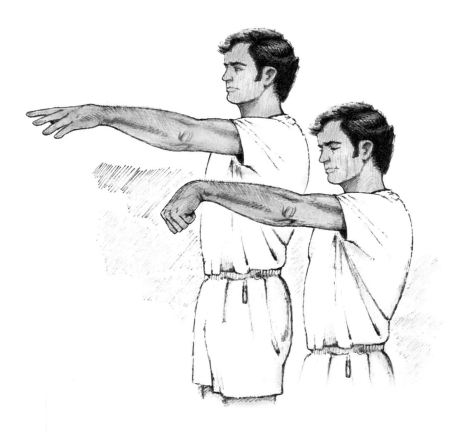

Finger Extensor
Starting position: Stand erect with your arm held out straight in front of you. Make a loose fist. Inhale. **Action:** While exhaling, curl your fist downward and assist with the opposite hand if necessary. Stretch to light irritation and hold for two seconds. Inhale while you return to the starting position. Repeat four to ten times, depending on your fitness level. Repeat for your other arm.

Hip and Leg Stretches

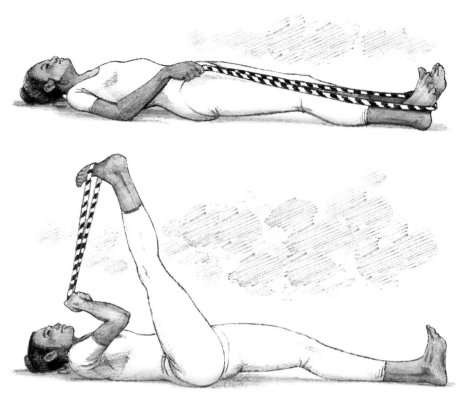

Straight Leg Hamstrings

Starting position: Lie flat on your back, legs straight, with a rope around the foot of the leg you will stretch. If you don't have a rope, you can use your hands to assist in this stretch. Keep your other leg flat on the floor. If you have a back problem, then use a cushion under the knee you aren't stretching. Inhale. **Action:** While exhaling, bring your straight leg toward your head until you feel tension. Use the rope to assist the stretch to light irritation and hold for two seconds. Inhale while you return to the starting position. Repeat four to ten times, depending on your fitness level. Repeat for your other leg.

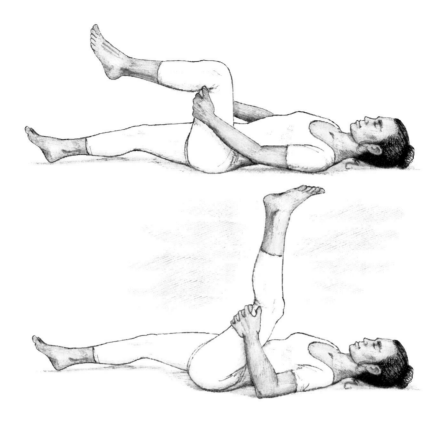

Bent Leg Hamstrings

Starting position: Lie flat on your back. Start with one knee bent to a 90-degree angle. Keep your other leg flat on the floor. If you have a back problem, use a cushion under the knee you aren't stretching. Inhale.
Action: While exhaling, bring your bent knee toward your chest. You can use your hands behind your thigh or a rope around your foot to assist the stretch. Straighten the leg, keeping the knee "soft." Stretch to light irritation and hold for two seconds. Inhale while you return to the starting position. Repeat four to ten times, depending on your fitness level. Repeat for your other leg.

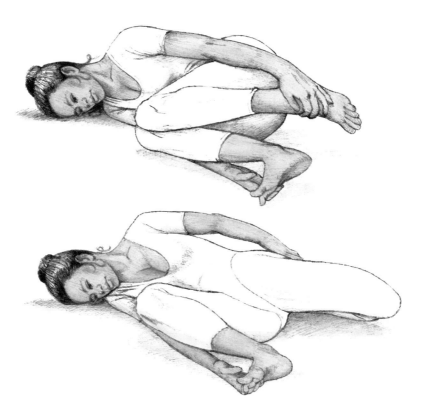

Quadriceps

Starting position: Lie on your side and bring the bottom knee close to your chest by holding the knee or foot. This will stabilize the low back to avoid strain. The top leg is your exercising leg. Bend the knee, keeping the leg level with the hip. Inhale. **Action:** While exhaling, bring your foot back toward your buttock. Use your hand or a rope on top of the foot and ankle of your upper leg to assist the movement. Stretch to light irritation and hold for two seconds. To increase the stretch, move the knee behind your body. Inhale while you return to the starting position. Repeat four to ten times, depending on your fitness level. Repeat for your other leg.

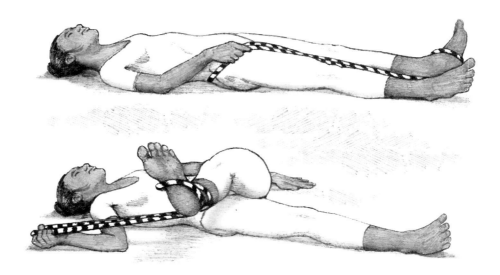

Tensor Fascia Latae (TFL)

Starting position: Lie flat on your back with your legs straight. Inhale.
Action: While exhaling, bring one leg over the opposite leg with the sole of the foot facing outward (eversion). Keep your buttock close to the floor with the leg low and as close to the nonexercising leg as possible. Assist with a rope around your ankle for a further stretch. Stretch to light irritation and hold for two seconds. Inhale while you return to the starting position. Repeat four to ten times, depending on your fitness level. Repeat for your other leg.

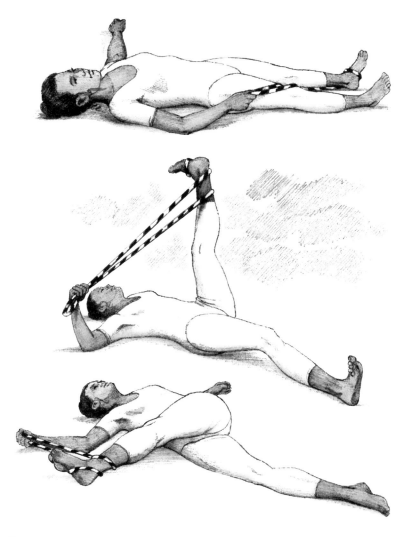

Figure Four

Starting position: Lie flat on your back with legs straight. Inhale.

Action: While exhaling, bring one straight leg up and across your body toward the floor. You can assist with a rope on your ankle for a further stretch. Keep your shoulders as close to the floor as possible and imagine leaving your buttocks behind. Stretch to light irritation and hold for two seconds. Inhale while you return to the starting position. Repeat four to ten times, depending on your fitness level. Repeat for your other leg.

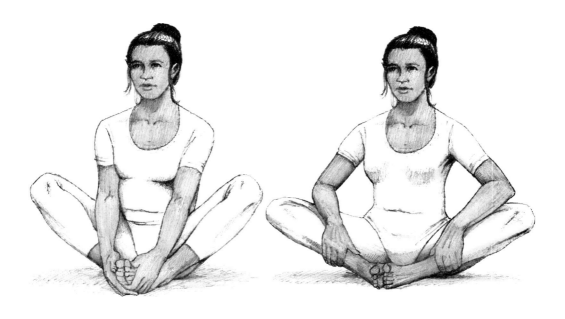

Adductors
Starting position: Sit on the floor with the soles of your feet together and your hands on your knees (stomach tucked, sternum up). Inhale.
Action: While exhaling, lower your knees toward the floor and hold for two seconds. Assist the stretch to light irritation by using your hands. Inhale while you return to the starting position. Repeat four to ten times, depending on your fitness level.

Trunk Stretches

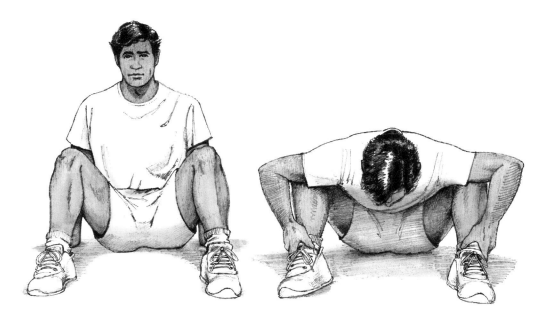

Forward Trunk Bend

Starting position: Sit erect on the floor with your knees bent. Your feet should be wider than shoulder width apart and flat on the floor. Inhale.

Action: While exhaling, contract your abdominal muscles, tuck your chin, and round your back as you roll forward between your legs. Assist by gently pulling on your ankles with your hands. Stretch to light irritation and hold for two seconds. Inhale while you return to the starting position. Repeat four to ten times, depending on your fitness level.

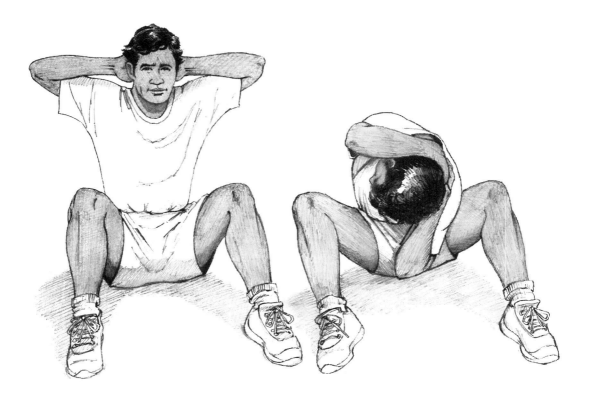

Twisting Trunk Bend

Starting position: Sit erect on the floor with your knees bent. Your feet should be wider than shoulder width apart and flat on the floor. Interlace your fingers behind your head. Inhale. **Action:** While exhaling, tuck your chin, twist your body to the right, and lower the right shoulder down between your legs. Contract the muscles on the side of your body to pull you down. Stretch to light irritation and hold for two seconds. Inhale while you return to the starting position. Repeat four to ten times, depending on your fitness level. Repeat on the other side.

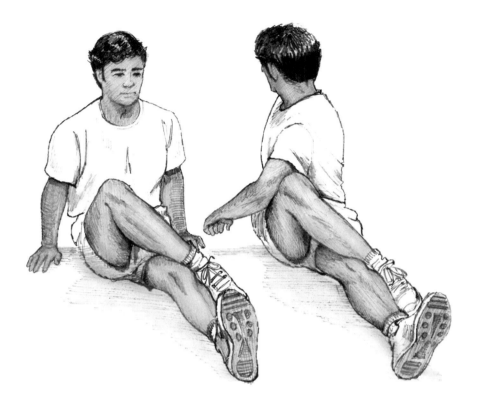

Spinal Twist

Starting position: Sit on the floor with your left leg straight out in front of you. Bend the right leg and cross it over your straight left leg. Inhale.

Action: While exhaling, turn your body to the right and look behind you. To assist this stretch, use your left elbow to gently push against the right knee. Stretch to light irritation and hold for two seconds. Inhale while you return to the starting position. Repeat four to ten times, depending on your fitness level. Repeat on the other side. Note: Experiment with the position of your elbow on your knee to affect the stretch.

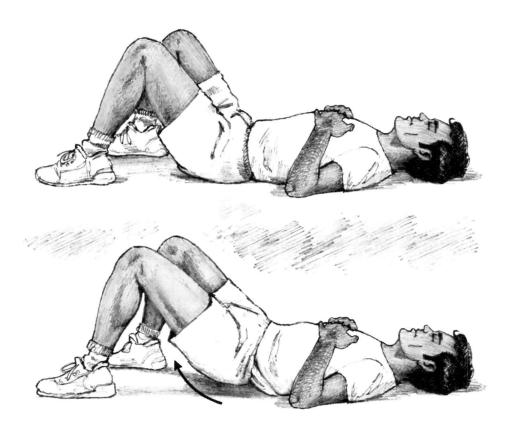

Pelvic Tilt

Starting position: Lie flat on your back with both knees bent, feet flat on the floor. Inhale. **Action:** While exhaling, contract your lower abdominals to roll your pelvis up so that the low back is flat and the distance between pelvis and navel is shortened. Stretch to light irritation and hold for two seconds. Inhale while you return to the starting position. Repeat four to ten times, depending on your fitness level.

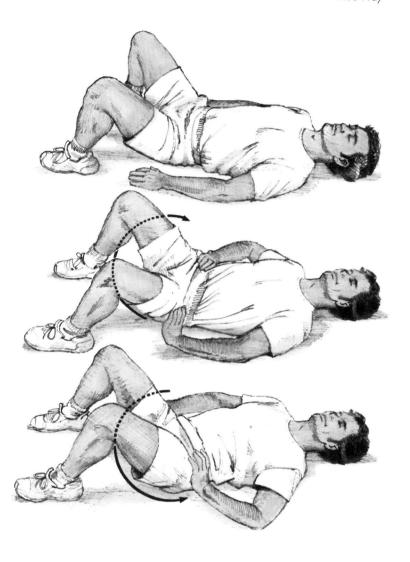

Hip Hiker

Starting position: Lie on your back with your knees bent and feet flat. Place your hands on your hips and inhale. **Action:** While exhaling, stretch one hip downward toward your foot. Glide the other hip up toward your shoulder using your hands to assist with further stretch. Stretch to light irritation and hold for two seconds. Inhale while you return to the starting position. Repeat four to ten times, depending on your fitness level. Repeat on the other side.

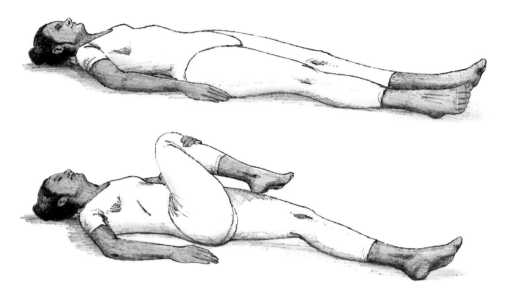

Knee to Opposite Shoulder

Starting position: Lie flat on your back with your legs straight. Inhale.
Action: While exhaling, bring one knee toward the opposite shoulder. Assist with your hand on your knee for a further stretch. Keep your hip as close to the floor as possible. Imagine you are going to leave those buttocks behind on the floor as your knee moves toward your shoulder. Stretch to light irritation and hold for two seconds. Inhale while you return to the starting position. Repeat four to ten times, depending on your fitness level. Repeat for your other leg.

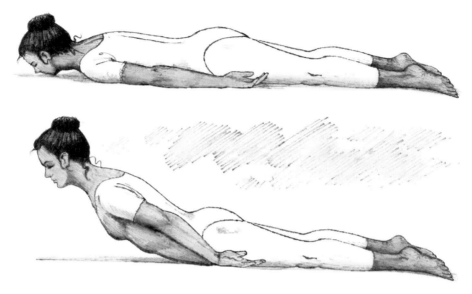

Thoracic Lift

Starting position: Lie face down with your arms at your sides. Inhale.
Action: While exhaling, flatten your pelvis to the floor, contract your
buttocks muscles, and lift your shoulders and chest off the floor. Stretch to
light irritation and hold for two seconds. Inhale while you return to the
starting position. Repeat four to ten times, depending on your fitness level.
Note: As with any exercise involving the spine, if you experience any active
or acute discomfort or pain or if you have a known disk problem, check with
your health care provider before doing this stretch.

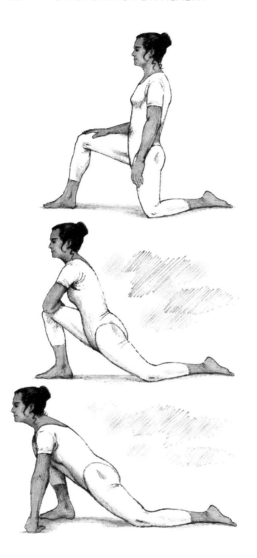

Iliopsoas

Starting position: Kneel on one knee. The other knee is bent and stays at a 90-degree angle in front of you with your foot flat on the floor. Inhale. **Action:** While exhaling, lean forward into your hip. You should feel a stretch in the upper leg and pelvis. Stretch to light irritation and hold for two seconds. Inhale while you return to the starting position. Repeat four to ten times, depending on your fitness level. Repeat on the other side. For a more advanced stretch, turn your head toward the side with the knee bent.

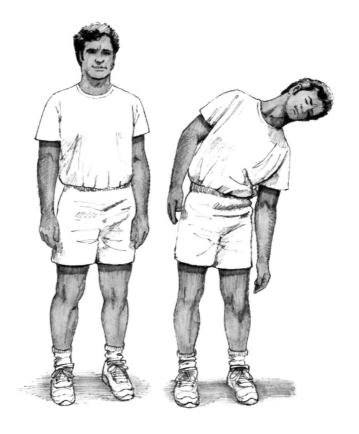

Side Bends

Starting position: Stand with your body erect and in good alignment, arms hanging at your sides. Inhale. **Action:** While exhaling, bend to one side so that your fingertips move closer to that knee. Stretch to light irritation and hold for two seconds. Inhale while you return to the starting position. Repeat four to ten times, depending on your fitness level. Repeat on the other side. For a more advanced side bend stretch, as the fingertips of one hand move toward the knee, bring the opposite arm over your head.

Lower Leg Stretches

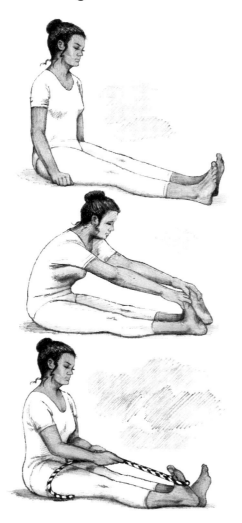

Calf Stretch–Gastrocnemius
Starting position: Sit on the floor with both legs straight in front of you. Inhale. **Action:** While exhaling, keep the legs straight and bring your toes toward your knees to stretch the back of your calf. You can assist with your hands or a rope around your foot to further the stretch. Stretch to light irritation and hold for two seconds. Inhale while you return to the starting position. Repeat four to ten times, depending on your fitness level. Repeat for your other leg.

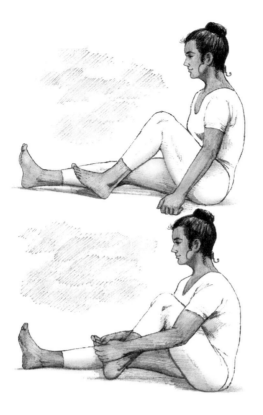

Soleus

Starting position: Sit on the floor and bring one knee up into a bent position. Inhale. **Action:** While exhaling, hold the ball of your foot with both hands and bring your toes toward you, assisting with your hands into a further stretch if necessary. Stretch to light irritation and hold for two seconds. Inhale while you return to the starting position. Repeat four to ten times, depending on your fitness level. Repeat for your other leg.

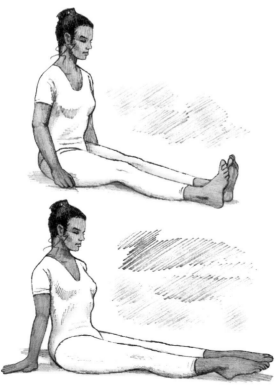

Tibialis Anterior

Starting position: Sit on the floor with both legs straight. Inhale. **Action:** While exhaling, point your toes away from your body to stretch the front of your lower leg. Stretch to light irritation and hold for two seconds. Inhale while you return to the starting position. Repeat four to ten times, depending on your fitness level. Repeat for the other leg.

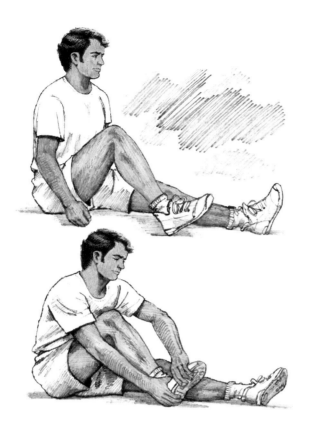

Eversion
(stretches the invertors)
Starting position: Sit on the
floor and bring one knee up
to a bent position. Inhale.
Action: While exhaling, bring
the sole of your foot toward
the outside and up. Assist
with your hands for a further
stretch. Stretch to light irritation and hold for two
seconds. Inhale while you
return to the starting
position. Repeat four to ten
times, depending on your fitness level. Repeat for your
other leg.

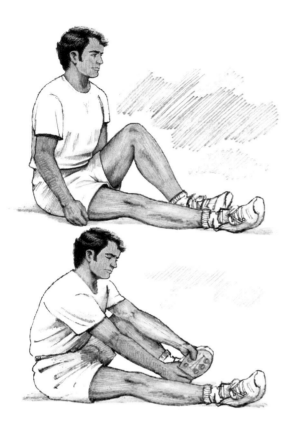

Inversion
(stretches the evertors)

Starting position: Sit on the floor and bring one knee up to a bent position. Inhale.
Action: While exhaling, bring the sole of your foot to the inside. Assist with your hands for a further stretch. Stretch to light irritation and hold for two seconds. Inhale while you return to the starting position. Repeat four to ten times, depending on your fitness level. Repeat for your other leg.

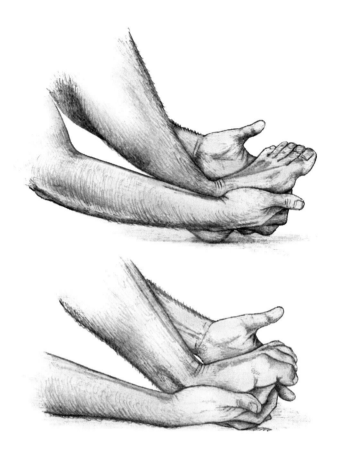

Metatarsal (good for hammer toes, bunions, and plantar fasciitis)
Starting position: Sit with one knee bent and the ankle in a flexed position with the fingers of both hands under the ball of your foot. Inhale.
Action: While exhaling, curl your toes around your fingers and stretch downward. Stretch to light irritation and hold for two seconds. Inhale while you return to the starting position. Repeat four to ten times, depending on your fitness level.

Questions and Answers

Q. I don't feel anything when I stretch. What does this mean?

A. You may want to change the angle at which you are stretching. Try to identify and isolate the area you wish to stretch. It also may mean that particular muscle is already flexible. We suggest you continue the movement anyway for balance and symmetry.

Q. I am large breasted and am not able to reach across my chest and feel a stretch. Any suggestions?

A. A prop may be necessary. We suggest you stand in front of the wall. With your forearm near shoulder height, place your upper arm on the wall just above the elbow. Carefully lean your body weight into the wall.

Q. I feel a pinch in the front of my shoulder when I reach across my chest to stretch the back of my shoulder. Why?

A. This may indicate that other muscles may need to be stretched before trying this stretch.

Q. Does stretching need to hurt to do any good?

A. No. There should not be any pain while stretching. Pain is an indicator that something needs to change. This may mean changing the angle of your stretching or the intensity of your routine. We suggest that stretching be taken only to light irritation.

Q. What do you mean by stretching to "light irritation"?

A. This is stretching to the point where a slight tug is felt. We often use the concept of "ah, it hurts so good." Again, if pain is felt, the intensity, angle, or particular stretch needs to change.

Q. What is the noise I hear in or around my joints while I move or stretch?

A. These noises are commonly referred to as crepitus and popping. They can be due to a number of things and there are varying opinions about what causes them. The most likely reasons are as follows:

- The noise is a result of tissue repair. Throughout daily activities, we incur microtears of the soft tissue. The healing process leaves a surface that is roughened and fibrotic, and the tissues are no longer able to glide smoothly.
- There may be a calcification of the soft tissue attachments around the joint.
- It could indicate that the articulating surfaces of the joint are worn, and what you hear is bone on bone grinding.

- Popping or snapping sounds could indicate a tendon or ligament moving over a bony prominence.

None of these is serious in and of themselves, and appropriate stretching can actually benefit. If any of these symptoms is accompanied by acute and lasting pain, seek advice from your health care provider.

Q. Is it true that people become less flexible as they get older? I've been told it's just my age and there's nothing else I can do.

A. Flexibility decreases with lack of use. Age combined with a history of inactivity means that the process of becoming flexible may take longer and more caution must be used. However, it's never too late to begin. For more on aging and fitness, see Chapter 5.

Glossary

Abduction movement away from the midline of the body

Adduction movement toward the midline of the body

Aerobic use of oxygen as the source of energy; by which an organism can live only in the presence of oxygen

Aerobic exercise involving or improving oxygen consumption by the body

Agonist muscle a muscle that is the prime mover and is opposed in action by another muscle called the antagonist; when the agonist contracts, its opposite, the antagonist relaxes

Amino acids 22 different amino acids are required to build all the proteins needed by the body; many of the amino acids necessary in metabolism can be synthesized in the human or animal body when needed and are called nonessential; others cannot be synthesized in sufficient quantities, are termed essential, and must be provided in the diet

Analgesics pain relievers such as aspirin, ibuprofen, and nonsteroidal antiin-flammatory drugs (NSAIDs)

Antagonist muscle refers to a muscle working in opposition to the action of another muscle called the agonist

Atherosclerosis hardening of the arteries (arteriosclerosis) due to plaques containing fatty substances (cholesterol and lipids) deposited on the innermost layer of the walls of arteries restricting blood flow

Autoimmune disease a disease that attacks the body's immune system and lowers its natural defenses

Biomechanics proper posture, proper lifting, and proper movement patterns

Body mechanics efficient use of body posture in relation to the activity being performed to prevent injury and maintain stamina

Cardiovascular pertaining to the heart and blood vessels of the body

Carpal tunnel syndrome a condition related to overuse of the arm and shoulder resulting in pain and often numbness and swelling in the wrist area; carpal refers to the carpal bones of the wrist; tunnel refers to the small tunnellike area where the tendons, nerves, and blood vessels pass through

Chelated a process whereby a bonding occurs to allow better absorption of nutrients; not to be confused with chelation therapy, which aids the elimination of toxic substances

Chemotherapeutic agents potent medications used in the treatment of cancer and severe forms of arthritis

Coenzymes necessary to assist enzymes in the completion of their action, as in digestion

Complementary medicine (integrative medicine) medicine other than modern western or allopathic medicine; some examples would be naturopathic medicine, homeopathic medicine, acupuncture, massage therapy, and oriental bodyworks such as shiatsu and jin shin

Contraindicated not a recommended procedure or medication for the symptoms displayed

Correct posture imaginary line running straight through the body (while standing): sternum is raised up, stomach is tucked, and feet are facing forward, shoulder-width apart and flat on the floor

Corticosteroids a class of medications that reduces inflammation and may have significant side effects

Cumulative trauma disorder damage to the soft tissue that has occurred over a prolonged period of time

Deconditioning a change that takes place in the cardiovascular, neuromuscular, and metabolic functions as a result of prolonged bed rest or inactivity

Dehydration a condition due to excessive loss of water from the body or from an organ or a body part, as from illness or lack of fluids

Dynamic characterized by continuous change, activity, or progress

Dynamic sitting sitting with frequent change of positions and movement of various joints

Electrolytes any of various ions, such as sodium, potassium, or chloride, required by cells to regulate the electric charge and flow of water molecules across the cell membrane

Ergonomics the science of examining and adapting the work environment to the individual's needs to reduce work-related musculoskeletal disorders

Essential amino acids a group of eight amino acids that are not easily synthesized by the body and must be supplied through diet

Eversion to turn or rotate (the hand or forearm) so that the palm faces down or back or to turn or rotate (the sole of the foot) by abduction and eversion so that the inner edge of the sole bears the body's weight; also known as pronation

Extension straightening or extending a limb using the extensor muscles

Flexion The act of bending a joint or limb in the body using the flexor muscles

Free radical An organic compound in which some of the valence electrons are unpaired, which promotes cell mutation and premature aging

Good alignment see *Correct posture*

Hydration the act of supplying water to restore or maintain fluid balance

Immune system the body's natural defense system

Immunostimulants medications that enhance or stimulate the immune system

Intervertebral disk a substance that functions like a shock absorber between vertebrae of the spine

Inversion to turn (the foot or leg) so that the sole is inward with the outer edge of the foot bearing weight; to supinate

Ischemia a decrease in the blood supply and oxygen to a bodily organ, tissue, or part caused by constriction or obstruction of the blood vessels

Isotonic of or involving muscular contraction in which the muscle remains under relatively constant tension while its length changes

Kinetic of, relating to, or produced by motion

Lateral movement away from the midline, or part of the body farther away from the midline

Lipids a similar group of fats and related substances that are insoluble in water but soluble in organic solvents; lipids are easily stored in the body, serve as a source of fuel, are an important part of cell structure, and serve other biological functions; major classes of lipids include fatty acids, neutral fats, waxes, and steroids; lipids are further defined as high density lipids (HDL—good cholesterol) and low density lipids (LDL—bad cholesterol)

Medial movement toward the midline, or part of the body closest to midline

Metabolic waste product a product of the body's metabolism that is no longer of benefit and is eliminated through organs such as the kidneys, liver, lungs, and intestines

Metabolism sum of all living processes in living systems; the process by which nutrients are absorbed and waste products eliminated

Midline while standing in correct posture, this is the imaginary line that divides your body into left and right. It runs down through the nose, through the navel, and down to the floor

Muscle spasm acute—a sudden involuntary contraction of a muscle or group of muscles accompanied by pain and interference of action; chronic—a prolonged contraction of a muscle that may feel like a knot and often results in pain

Muscle sprain overstretching or overuse that may result in tearing of soft tissue such as ligaments

Muscle strain stress or tear to soft tissue such as tendon and muscle; tends to occur from repetitive use or repeated trauma; usually less severe than a sprain

Musculoskeletal the soft tissue and bones in the body

Musculotendinous pertaining to the muscles and tendon attachments

Neuritis inflammation of a nerve or group of nerves, characterized by pain, loss of reflexes, and atrophy of the affected muscles

Neutral position comfortable posture, with joints naturally aligned to reduce musculoskeletal disorders

Nodule in relation to arthritis, it can be a benign overgrowth of calcium or lump within or near a joint

Overuse syndrome see *Cumulative trauma disorder*

Pain a more or less localized sensation of discomfort resulting from stimulation of specialized nerve endings; pain serves as a protective mechanism in that it prompts the individual to remove or withdraw from the source

Pronation to turn or rotate (the hand or forearm) so that the palm faces down or back; to turn or rotate (the sole of the foot) by abduction and eversion so that the inner edge of the sole bears the body's weight

Proper posture see *Correct posture*

Protein synthesis the process by which proteins (amino acids) are formed by normal body metabolism

Reciprocal inhibition a theory stating that if one muscle or muscle group is contracted, then the opposing muscle or muscle group must relax (inhibit)

Reciprocal innervation a theory stating that if one muscle or muscle group is relaxed, then the opposing muscle or muscle group must contract (innervate) to produce an action

Repetitive stress injury see *Cumulative trauma disorder*

Rheumatologist a physician specializing in the treatment of arthritis and conditions involving inflammation

Rheumatology pertaining to inflammation, soreness, and stiffness of joints and muscles

Rotator cuff muscles a group of four muscles that surround the shoulder joint holding the humerus (upper arm) in place and allow for circumduction or a 360-degree range of motion of the arm: the supraspinatus, infraspinatus, teres minor, and subscapularis

Scapula shoulder blade

Soft elbow slightly flexed or bent

Soft knee slightly flexed or bent

Soft tissue general term referring to soft structures such as muscles, tendons, or ligaments

Spasm see *Muscle spasm*

Sternum breastbone

Stretch to light irritation stretch until a light tug is felt or until it "hurts so good"

Stretch weakness the weakening of muscles that are habitually kept stretched beyond their normal resting state; for example, cradling the telephone to your ear for an extended period of time, on a daily basis

Supination to turn (the hand and forearm) so that the palm is upward or forward, or to turn (the foot or leg) so that the sole is inward

Supine lying face up

Sustained posture posture that is held for a long period of time and requires muscle contraction to hold that position; when the muscles remain contracted, the blood flow and circulation to the muscle is reduced and chance of injury is increased

Synthesize to combine substances so as to form a new, complex product

Target heart rate the heart rate range during exercise that can produce maximum aerobic benefit to the heart and lungs, usually 60 to 85 percent of maximum capacity

Tendinitis the inflammation of tendons and tendon-muscle attachments due to chronic repetitive motion; it may result in scarring or calcium deposits in a tendon, and pain and/or loss of range of motion can also occur

Thoracic outlet syndrome a condition where a nerve and/or blood vessel may be pinched or occluded in the shoulder area with resulting pain and numbness down the arm

Trans fatty acids lipids that are believed to be more harmful than saturated fats or excessive cholesterol; they are present in polyunsaturated fats (when exposed to air and expecially when heated) and hydrogenated fats or oils

Vertebral disks gelatinous structures between the vertebrae that act like cushions, preventing bone from rubbing on bone

References

Alter, Michael J. 1988. *Science of stretching*. Champaign, Illinois: Human Kinetics Books.

Balch, James, and Phyllis Balch. 1992. *Prescription for cooking and dietary wellness*. Greenfield, Indiana: PAB books.

Balch, James, and Phyllis Balch. 1990. *Prescription for nutritional healing*. Garden City Park, New York: Avery Publication Group.

Benson, Hubert, and Eileen Stuart. 1992. *The wellness book*. New York: Simon and Schuster/Fireside Books.

Center for Science in the Public Interest. 1992–1996. *Nutrition Action Health Letter*. Washington, D. C.

Chaitow, Leon. 1990. *The body/mind purification program*. New York: Simon and Schuster/Fireside Books.

Conn, Doyt L. 1997. Most asked questions. *Arthritis Today* (January–February).

Ford, Norman D. 1997. *18 natural ways to stop arthritis now*. New Canaan, Connecticut: Keats Publishing.

Gittleman, Ann Louise. 1999. *Eat fat, lose weight*. New Canaan, Connecticut: Keats Publishing.

Hebert, Lauren Andrew. 1989. *The neck-arm-hand book: The master guide for eliminating cumulative trauma disorders from the workplace*. Bangor, Maine. IMPACC.

Kirschmann, John. 1979. *Nutrition Almanac*. New York: McGraw-Hill Book Company.

Knight, E. Leslie, and Aaron L. Mattes. 1998. *Nutrition therapy for massage and physical therapy patients*. Sarasota, Florida: Aaron L. Mattes, M.S., R.K.T., L.M.T.

Mattes, Aaron L., 1995. *Active isolated stretching*. Sarasota, Florida: Aaron L. Mattes, M.S., R.K.T., L.M.T.

Mattes, Aaron L., 1980. *Flexibility, active and assisted stretching*. Sarasota, Florida: Aaron L. Mattes, M.S., R.K.T., L.M.T.

Mattes, Aaron L., 1980. *Flexibility for conditioning and rehabilitation*. Sarasota, Florida: Aaron L. Mattes, M.S., R.K.T., L.M.T.

McClary, Cheryl, and Keith Ray. 1994. *Wellness and the liberal arts*. Dubuque, Iowa: Kendall/Hunt Publication.

Riggs, Gail Kershner. 1997. A patient's/health professional's historical and hysterical 50 year perspective of arthritis. Paper presented at lecture, University of Arizona Medical School, Tucson, Arizona.

Ryan, Regina, and John Travis. 1981. *Wellness workbook*. 1981. Berkeley, California: Ten Speed Press.

Shelton, Robert E., Leonard O. Greninger, and Aaron L. Mattes. 1973. *Basic exercise, pre-conditioning and re-habilitation*. Dubuque, Iowa: Eddie Bowers Publishing Company.

INDEX

British Guidelines on the Management of Acute Back Pain, 54

Bursitis, 48

Caffeine, 20, 31

Calcium, 16

Carbohydrates, 11
  simple vs. complex, 11
  unrefined vs. refined, 11

Carbonated beverages, 20, 31

Cardiac rehabilitation exercise, 68

Cardiovascular, 116

Carpal tunnel syndrome, 24–25, 26, 50–52, 116
  aggravating factors, 51
  definition, 50–51
  self-help measures, 52
  stretching recommendations, 52

Checkout persons, 25, 72

Chelated, 116

Chemotherapeutic agents, 116

Child, Julia, 18

Cholesterol, 12, 13–14
  LDL vs. HDL, 14

Chronic fatigue syndrome, 37–39
  aggravating factors, 38
  definition, 37–38
  energy conservation and, 38–39
  self-help measures, 38–39
  stretching recommendations, 38–39

Coenzymes, 16, 116

Complementary medicine, 116

Computer work, 27–28, 71

Contraindicated procedure, 116

Control of life, 2

Cooldown exercises, 61

Corticosteroids, 116

Cumulative trauma disorder, 24–27, 116
  factors that contribute to, 29

Cycling, 71

Deconditioning, 116

Dehydration, 20, 31, 116

Diet. *See* Nutrition

Digestion, 10

Driving, 71

Dynamic, 116

Dynamic sitting, 116

Dysfunctional biomechanics, 44

Eating. *See* Food

Electrolyte replacement, 20

Electrolytes, 116

Enriched food, 17

Ergonomics, 26–27, 41, 117

Essential amino acids, 117

Essential fatty acids (EFAS), 13

Eversion, 117

Exercising. *See also specific body parts*
  active-isolated method, 60, 62, 69–114
  aerobic exercising, 7, 30, 39, 64–67
  arthritis and, 35
  cooldown, 61
  fluid replacement and, 20–21
  questions and answers, 113–14
  warm-up exercises, 27, 61

Extension, 117

Fats, 11–14
  absorption of vitamins and, 11
  foods with, 13
  good, 13

Fatty acid
  saturated vs. unsaturated, 12

Fibromyalgia syndrome, 37–39

Finger exercise
  finger extensor, 92
  finger flexor, 91

Flexibility, 1, 59–64. *See also* Stretching
  active-isolated method, 60, 62, 69–114
  age and, 68, 114

About the Authors

Jerry Weinert is a registered nurse, certified neuromuscular therapist, certified instructor of Thai medical massage (Nuad Bo-Rarn), and is nationally certified in therapeutic massage and bodywork. For over fifteen years, Jerry has been actively involved with rehabilitation, wellness counseling, and flexibility training for adults of all ages. While living in Asheville, North Carolina, he served as the Program Director of Heart Path, a multiple-intervention cardiac rehabilitation program, directed the Thoms Rehabilitation Hospital Outpatient Center, and founded and directed the Integrated Health Consultants, a group of complementary health care practitioners. He served as Vice President of the Buncombe County Unit of the American Heart Association and was on the Board of the Western North Carolina Minority Health Program. Jerry currently lives and works in Tucson, Arizona. In addition to his private practice, he has been on the faculty of Phoenix Therapeutic Massage College and is currently a faculty member at the Desert Institute of the Healing Arts. Jerry is a professional member of the American Massage Therapy Association, the National Association of Nurse Massage Therapists, and the International Association of Healthcare Practitioners. He has been the State Representative for the National Association of Nurse Massage Therapists in North Carolina and Arizona and recently completed a three-year term on the Board of Directors for National Certification Board for Therapeutic Massage and Bodywork. Jerry is codirector of Southwest Wellness Educators.

Jill Bielawski has been a practicing, licensed massage therapist in Tucson, Arizona, for over thirteen years. She is nationally certified in therapeutic massage and bodywork and is a member of the national sports massage team. Jill also holds certificates in myofascial therapy and in the oriental bodywork modalities of Shiatsu and Tuina. She was an instructor of sports massage at the Desert Institute of the Healing Arts in Tucson, Arizona, for six years and during that time gained affiliation for the program with the University of Arizona training room. Jill was employed by the University of Arizona Swim

Team for several years and traveled to major meets including those of the PAC 10, NCAA, and Olympic Trials. She is currently in private practice and specializes in deep, specific massage and pain management. She is the former Director of Education for the Arizona chapter of the American Massage Therapy Association and served as editor of the chapter newsletter, receiving state and national awards. Jill is codirector of Southwest Wellness Educators. Jill holds a Bachelor of Science degree in vocational rehabilitation from the University of Arizona and has worked with hearing-impaired and multiple-handicapped children. She is the first Western woman known to have trekked through the deepest valley of the world, Namche Barwa, in Eastern Tibet.

Southwestern Wellness Educators is dedicated to providing current and ongoing education of wellness and flexibility. Individual instruction and group workshops are available. Topics include flexibility, body mechanics, workplace ergonomics, and overuse injury prevention.